INFORMATION NEEDS AND CHALLENGES IN CANCER RESEARCH

Workshop Summary

Sharyl J. Nass and Theresa Wizemann, *Rapporteurs*

National Cancer Policy Forum
Board on Health Care Services

INSTITUTE OF MEDICINE
OF THE NATIONAL ACADEMIES

THE NATIONAL ACADEMIES PRESS
Washington, D.C.
www.nap.edu

THE NATIONAL ACADEMIES PRESS   500 Fifth Street, NW   Washington, DC 20001

NOTICE: The project that is the subject of this report was approved by the Governing Board of the National Research Council, whose members are drawn from the councils of the National Academy of Sciences, the National Academy of Engineering, and the Institute of Medicine.

This study was supported by Contract Nos. HHSN261200900003C and 200-2005-13434 TO #1 between the National Academy of Sciences and the National Cancer Institute and the Centers for Disease Control and Prevention, respectively. In addition, the National Cancer Policy Forum is supported by the American Association for Cancer Research, the American Cancer Society, the American Society of Clinical Oncology, the Association of American Cancer Institutes, Bristol-Myers Squibb, C-Change, the CEO Roundtable on Cancer, Novartis Oncology, and the Oncology Nursing Society. The views presented in this publication do not necessarily reflect the view of the organizations or agencies that provided support for this project.

International Standard Book Number-13:   978-0-309-25948-4
International Standard Book Number-10:   0-309-25948-7

Additional copies of this report are available from the National Academies Press, 500 Fifth Street, NW, Keck 360, Washington, DC 20001; (800) 624-6242 or (202) 334-3313; http://www.nap.edu.

For more information about the Institute of Medicine, visit the IOM home page at: **www.iom.edu.**

Copyright 2012 by the National Academy of Sciences. All rights reserved.

Printed in the United States of America

Cover credit: Design by Casey Weeks.

The serpent has been a symbol of long life, healing, and knowledge among almost all cultures and religions since the beginning of recorded history. The serpent adopted as a logotype by the Institute of Medicine is a relief carving from ancient Greece, now held by the Staatliche Museen in Berlin.

Suggested citation: IOM (Institute of Medicine). 2012. *Informatics needs and challenges in cancer research: Workshop summary.* Washington, DC: The National Academies Press.

*"Knowing is not enough; we must apply.
Willing is not enough; we must do."*
—Goethe

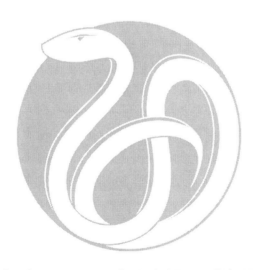

INSTITUTE OF MEDICINE
OF THE NATIONAL ACADEMIES

Advising the Nation. Improving Health.

THE NATIONAL ACADEMIES
Advisers to the Nation on Science, Engineering, and Medicine

The **National Academy of Sciences** is a private, nonprofit, self-perpetuating society of distinguished scholars engaged in scientific and engineering research, dedicated to the furtherance of science and technology and to their use for the general welfare. Upon the authority of the charter granted to it by the Congress in 1863, the Academy has a mandate that requires it to advise the federal government on scientific and technical matters. Dr. Ralph J. Cicerone is president of the National Academy of Sciences.

The **National Academy of Engineering** was established in 1964, under the charter of the National Academy of Sciences, as a parallel organization of outstanding engineers. It is autonomous in its administration and in the selection of its members, sharing with the National Academy of Sciences the responsibility for advising the federal government. The National Academy of Engineering also sponsors engineering programs aimed at meeting national needs, encourages education and research, and recognizes the superior achievements of engineers. Dr. Charles M. Vest is president of the National Academy of Engineering.

The **Institute of Medicine** was established in 1970 by the National Academy of Sciences to secure the services of eminent members of appropriate professions in the examination of policy matters pertaining to the health of the public. The Institute acts under the responsibility given to the National Academy of Sciences by its congressional charter to be an adviser to the federal government and, upon its own initiative, to identify issues of medical care, research, and education. Dr. Harvey V. Fineberg is president of the Institute of Medicine.

The **National Research Council** was organized by the National Academy of Sciences in 1916 to associate the broad community of science and technology with the Academy's purposes of furthering knowledge and advising the federal government. Functioning in accordance with general policies determined by the Academy, the Council has become the principal operating agency of both the National Academy of Sciences and the National Academy of Engineering in providing services to the government, the public, and the scientific and engineering communities. The Council is administered jointly by both Academies and the Institute of Medicine. Dr. Ralph J. Cicerone and Dr. Charles M. Vest are chair and vice chair, respectively, of the National Research Council.

www.national-academies.org

WORKSHOP PLANNING COMMITTEE[1]

SHARON B. MURPHY (*Chair*), Scholar-in-Residence, National Cancer Policy Forum, Board on Health Care Services, Institute of Medicine, Washington, DC
AMY P. ABERNETHY (*Co-Vice Chair*), Associate Professor of Medicine, Division of Medical Oncology, Department of Medicine, Duke University School of Medicine; Director, Duke Cancer Care Research Program, Durham, NC
MARCIA KEAN (*Co-Vice Chair*), Chair, Strategic Initiatives, Feinstein Kean Healthcare, Cambridge, MA
ADAM CLARK, Patient Advocacy Consultant; Founder, MedTran Health Strategies, Washington, DC
WILLIAM S. DALTON, CEO, M2Gen Personalized Medicine Institute, Moffitt Cancer Center & Research Institute, University of South Florida, Tampa
BRADLEY H. POLLOCK, Professor and Chair, Henry B. Dielmann Distinguished University Chair, Department of Epidemiology and Biostatistics, School of Medicine, University of Texas Health Science Center at San Antonio
LAWRENCE N. SHULMAN, Chief Medical Officer and Senior Vice President for Medical Affairs and Chief, Division of General Oncology, Dana-Farber Cancer Institute, Boston, MA

Project Staff

ERIN BALOGH, Associate Program Officer
PAMELA LIGHTER, Research Assistant
MICHAEL PARK, Senior Program Assistant
SHARYL J. NASS, Director, National Cancer Policy Forum
ROGER HERDMAN, Director, Board on Health Care Services

---

[1] Institute of Medicine planning committees are solely responsible for organizing the workshop, identifying topics, and choosing speakers. The responsibility for the published workshop summary rests with the workshop rapporteurs and the institution.

NATIONAL CANCER POLICY FORUM[1]

JOHN MENDELSOHN (*Chair*), Co-Director, Khalifa Institute for Personalized Cancer Therapy, M.D. Anderson Cancer Center, Houston, TX

PATRICIA A. GANZ (*Vice-Chair*), Professor, University of California, Los Angeles, School of Medicine & Public Health, Division of Cancer Prevention & Control Research, Jonsson Comprehensive Cancer Center

AMY P. ABERNETHY, Associate Professor of Medicine, Duke University School of Medicine, and Director, Duke Cancer Care Research Program, Durham, NC

FRED APPELBAUM, Director, Clinical Research Division, Fred Hutchinson Cancer Research Center, Seattle, WA

PETER B. BACH, Attending Physician, Memorial Sloan-Kettering Cancer Center, New York, NY

EDWARD BENZ, JR., President, Dana-Farber Cancer Institute, and Director, Harvard Cancer Center, Harvard Medical School, Boston, MA

MONICA BERTAGNOLLI, Professor of Surgery, Harvard Medical School, Boston, MA

OTIS BRAWLEY, Chief Medical Officer and Executive Vice President, American Cancer Society, Atlanta, GA

MICHAEL A. CALIGIURI, Director, Ohio State Comprehensive Cancer Center, Columbus, and Past President, Association of American Cancer Institutes

RENZO CANETTA, Vice President, Oncology Global Clinical Research, Bristol-Myers Squibb, Wallingford, CT

MICHAELE CHAMBLEE CHRISTIAN, Retired, Washington, DC

WILLIAM DALTON, CEO, M2Gen Personalized Medicine Institute, Moffitt Cancer Center, Tampa, FL, and Chair, American Association for Cancer Research Science Policy & Legislative Affairs Committee

WENDY DEMARK-WAHNEFRIED, Associate Director for Cancer Prevention and Control, University of Alabama at Birmingham Comprehensive Cancer Center

ROBERT ERWIN, President, Marti Nelson Cancer Foundation, Davis, CA

ROY S. HERBST, Chief of Medical Oncology, Yale Cancer Center, New Haven, CT

---

[1] Institute of Medicine forums and roundtables do not issue, review, or approve individual documents. The responsibility for the published workshop summary rests with the workshop rapporteurs and the institution.

THOMAS J. KEAN, President and CEO, C-Change, Washington, DC
DOUGLAS R. LOWY, Deputy Director, National Cancer Institute, Bethesda, MD
DANIEL R. MASYS, Affiliate Professor, Biomedical Informatics, University of Washington, Seattle
MARTIN J. MURPHY, Chief Executive Officer, CEO Roundtable on Cancer, Durham, NC
BRENDA NEVIDJON, Clinical Professor and Specialty Director, Nursing & Healthcare Leadership, Duke University School of Nursing, Durham, NC, and Past President, Oncology Nursing Society
STEVEN PIANTADOSI, Director, Samuel Oschin Comprehensive Cancer Institute, Cedars-Sinai Medical Center, Los Angeles, CA
LISA C. RICHARDSON, Associate Director for Science, Division of Cancer Prevention and Control, Centers for Disease Control and Prevention, Atlanta, GA
YA-CHEN TINA SHIH, Director, Program in the Economics of Cancer, University of Chicago, IL
ELLEN SIGAL, Chairperson and Founder, Friends of Cancer Research, Washington, DC
STEVEN STEIN, Senior Vice President, U.S. Clinical Development and Medical Affairs, Novartis Oncology, East Hanover, NJ
JOHN A. WAGNER, Vice President, Clinical Pharmacology, Merck and Company, Inc., Rahway, NJ
RALPH R. WEICHSELBAUM, Chair, Radiation and Cellular Oncology, and Director, Ludwig Center for Metastasis Research, University of Chicago Medical Center, IL
JANET WOODCOCK, Director, Center for Drug Evaluation and Research, Food and Drug Administration, Rockville, MD

National Cancer Policy Forum Staff

SHARYL J. NASS, Director
LAURA LEVIT, Program Officer
ERIN BALOGH, Associate Program Officer
PAMELA LIGHTER, Research Assistant
MICHAEL PARK, Senior Program Assistant
PATRICK BURKE, Financial Associate
SHARON B. MURPHY, Scholar-in-Residence
ROGER HERDMAN, Director, Board on Health Care Services

Reviewers

This report has been reviewed in draft form by individuals chosen for their diverse perspectives and technical expertise, in accordance with procedures approved by the National Research Council's Report Review Committee. The purpose of this independent review is to provide candid and critical comments that will assist the institution in making its published report as sound as possible and to ensure that the report meets institutional standards for objectivity, evidence, and responsiveness to the study charge. The review comments and draft manuscript remain confidential to protect the integrity of the process. We wish to thank the following individuals for their review of this report:

GWEN DARIEN, Director, The Pathways Project
BRETT DAVIS, Senior Director, Strategy and Business Development, Oracle Health Sciences
CHARLES FRIEDMAN, Director, Health Informatics Program, Professor, Department of Health Management and Policy, Professor, School of Information, University of Michigan
MIA A. LEVY, Assistant Professor of Biomedical Informatics and Medicine, Vanderbilt University School of Medicine, Director, Cancer Clinical Informatics, Vanderbilt-Ingram Cancer Center

Although these reviewers have provided many constructive comments and suggestions, they did not see the final draft of the report before its release. The review of this report was overseen by **Melvin Worth.** Appointed by the Institute of Medicine, he was responsible for making certain that an independent examination of this report was carried out in accordance with institutional procedures and that all review comments were carefully considered. Responsibility for the final content of this report rests entirely with the rapporteurs and the institution.

Contents

1 **INTRODUCTION** 1
Organization of the Workshop and Summary, 4
References, 5

2 **OVERVIEW OF THE CANCER INFORMATICS LANDSCAPE** 7
Structured, Interoperable Research and Clinical Information Systems—Or the Lack Thereof, 8
  Data Overload, 8
  Databases That Foster Learning, 9
  Making Connections, 9
  Robust EHR Systems and Research Databases, 11
Cancer Center Informatics: Connecting with Patients, 12
  Research Information Exchange, 13
Cancer Cooperative Group Informatics: Connecting Researchers, 15
  Informatics Tools Used by the NCI Cooperative Group Program, 16
  Opportunities for an Innovative Informatics Structure, 17
Clinical Translational Research Informatics: Connecting the Steps of the Research Process, 18
  Hypothesis Driven Versus Hypothesis Generating, 19
  Study Design, 19

Informatics Challenges for Translational Research, 20
Moving Clinical Translational Informatics Forward, 22
caBIG—The Vision and the Reality, 22
    Looking Forward: A Three-Step Approach to Success in
        Informatics Innovation, 25
    Community Participation in Moving Informatics Forward, 28
References, 29

3   INFORMATICS AND PERSONALIZED MEDICINE   31
An Integrative Systems Approach to Biology, Medicine, and
        Complexity, 32
    Biology and Medicine as Informational Sciences, 33
    Systems Biology Infrastructure, 34
    Holistic Systems Experimental Approaches, 34
    Emerging Technologies, 37
    Domain-Driven, Transforming Analytic Tools, 39
Applications of Systems Medicine: The P4 Approach, 40
    Information Technology for Health Care, 40
References, 42

4   INFORMATICS-SUPPORTED CANCER RESEARCH
     ENDEAVORS   43
Case Example: Dell-TGen Cloud Computing Collaboration in
        Personalized Medicine for Pediatric Neuroblastoma, 44
    An $N = 1$ Approach to Clinical Research, 44
    Molecularly Guided Individualized Cancer Therapy, 46
    Opportunities in the Cloud, 47
Case Example: National Comprehensive Cancer Network Outcomes
        Database, 48
    NCCN Guidelines, 48
    NCCN Oncology Outcomes Database, 48
Case Example: IT Innovations for Community Cancer Practices, 51
    System Design and Datasets, 53
    Supporting Clinical Outcomes and Research, 54
    Data Governance, 54
Case Example: Secondary Uses of Data for Comparative Effectiveness
        Research, 54
    Secondary Use of Data, 56
    Sustainability, 57

CONTENTS   *xiii*

    Cross-Cutting Issues, 58
        Engaging Patients, 58
        Building Trust: Privacy, Consent, and Ownership, 58
        Data Granularity, 60
        Secondary Use, 60
        Engaging Private Practice and Extramural Researchers, 61
    References, 61

5   POTENTIAL PATHWAYS AND MODELS FOR MOVING FORWARD   63
    Public Data-Driven Systems and Personalized Medicine, 64
        Commoditization of Data, 64
        Integrative Genomics to Identify Novel Targets, 65
        Genomic Nosology and Drug or Diagnostic Discovery, 66
    Adapting to Data-Intensive, Data-Enabled Biomedicine, 67
        Data Production, Analysis, and Utilization in Biomedicine, 67
        Importance of Having the "Right" Data in the System, 69
        Computational Capabilities for Large Datasets, 70
        Moving from Silos to Systems, 72
    Big Data and Disruptive Innovation: Models for Democratizing Cancer Research and Care, 73
        Learning from Users of Big Data in Diverse Non-Health Venues, 74
        Disruptive Innovation, 76
        Democratizing Big Data Informatics for Cancer and Other Therapeutic Areas, 78
        Consumers as Disruptive Innovators, 81
    The EHR and Cancer Research and Care, 82
        Enhancing Uptake of EHRs, 82
        The EpicCare System as a Model for the Users of EHRs in Cancer Research and Care, 82
    Cancer Center–Based Networks for Health Research Information Exchange, 84
        Personalized Cancer Care, 84
        Proposed Federated Data Model, 86
    Other Models and Pathways, 86
        Patients Helping Patients, 87
        Providing a Substrate for Innovation, 87
        Mining Data to Assess the Quality of Cancer Care, 88

Fostering Sharing, 88
Education, Training, and Funding, 89
If Data Are Available, Users Will Come, 89
References, 89

6 PROPOSAL FOR A COALITION OF ALL STAKEHOLDERS   91
Achieving Data Liquidity in the Cancer Community, 91
Principles, 92
Operational Strategy and Activities, 92
Coalition Governance, Funding, and Sustainability, 93
Working Toward a National System, 94

7 TRANSFORMING CANCER INFORMATICS: FROM SILOS TO SYSTEMS   95
A Framework For Action, 97
Changing Minds, Changing Behaviors, 97

ACRONYMS   99

APPENDIXES

A   **Workshop Agenda**   103
B   **Speaker, Moderator, and Panelist Biographies**   109

Boxes, Figures, and Table

BOXES

2-1 Dana-Farber Synergistic Patient and Research Knowledge Systems (SPARKS), 11
2-2 Common Needs to Catalyze Effectiveness in Cancer Research That Helped to Shape the Priority Areas for the caBIG Activities, 23
2-3 NCI Informatics Project Review Criteria, 26

3-1 P4 Medicine: Perspectives from Leroy Hood on What the Future Could Hold, 41

4-1 What Real-World Data Are Used by Whom?, 52

6-1 Proposed Coalition Principles, 93

FIGURES

2-1 Rapid-learning health care system for cancer care, 10
2-2 Dana-Farber Synergistic Patient and Research Knowledge Systems (SPARKS), 12
2-3 Example of a research information exchange system at the Moffitt Cancer Center, integrating data from multiple sources and providing them to diverse stakeholders, 14

3-1 Systems biology infrastructure, 35
3-2 Systems medicine: A network of networks, 36

4-1 The evolution from evidence-based medicine to information-enabled medicine to intelligence-based medicine, 45

5-1 A new health care ecosystem arising from convergence of technologies and markets, 72
5-2 A new ecosystem of disruptive business models, 78
5-3 Learning health care paradigm supported by robust, interoperable informatics, 79
5-4 Designing a new federated research and health care network model, 84

7-1 Hypothetical framework highlighting key elements of an end-to-end cancer informatics system, 98

TABLE

4-1 The Evolving Evidence Perspective, 56

1

Introduction

Informatics tools are essential to biomedical and health research and development. The field of cancer research, like most scientific disciplines, is facing an overwhelming deluge of data that are increasingly challenging to collate, store, access, analyze, and exchange. There is a particular need to integrate research and clinical data to facilitate personalized medicine approaches to cancer prevention and treatment (e.g., tailoring treatment based on an individual patient's genetic makeup as well as that of the tumor) and to allow for more rapid learning from patient experiences (IOM, 2010, 2011). There is an increased national urgency to find solutions to support and sustain the cancer informatics ecosystem, especially in light of the recent devolution of the National Cancer Institute's (NCI's) Cancer Biomedical Informatics Grid® (caBIG) program.[1]

To further examine informatics[2] needs and challenges for 21st century biomedical research, the National Cancer Policy Forum of the Institute of

---

[1] caBIG is discussed further in Chapter 2. Note that caBIG and Cancer Biomedical Informatics Grid are registered trademarks.

[2] Biomedical informatics has been defined as the science that develops methods, techniques, and theories regarding how to use data, information, and knowledge to support and improve biomedical research, human health, and the delivery of health care services (http://www.amia.org/glossary). In the clinical arena, informatics is an applied and interdisciplinary field, at the intersection of information science, computer science, and clinical medicine, to provide improved patient care by harnessing and optimizing health information technology (Miriovsky et al., in press).

Medicine (IOM) held a public workshop[3] in Washington, DC, on February 27 and 28, 2012, using cancer research as a model research enterprise to consider the role of informatics from basic discovery science through translational research, product development, clinical trials, comparative effectiveness research, and health services research.

The workshop was designed to raise awareness of the critical and urgent importance of the challenges, gaps, and opportunities in informatics; to frame the issues surrounding the development of an integrated system of cancer informatics tools for acceleration of research; and to discuss solutions for transformation of the cancer informatics enterprise.

Specifically, invited speakers and participants considered the following:

- the design, development, and integration of informatics tools in cancer research;
- standards for cancer informatics tools;
- interoperability and harmonization;
- infrastructure needs for research;
- data annotation and curation of multiple complex datasets;
- methods for data use and representation;
- the implications of implementing effective informatics tools for research; and
- sustainability, governance, policy, and trust.

John Mendelsohn, co-director of the Khalifa Institute for Personalized Cancer Therapy at the University of Texas M.D. Anderson Cancer Center and chair of the IOM's National Cancer Policy Forum, stressed that informatics is much more than electronic health care records. He called upon participants to offer practical action items that could help to advance knowledge and improve informatics as applied to cancer research. An overview of key discussion points raised by individual presenters is provided here.

---

[3] This workshop was organized by an independent planning committee whose role was limited to the identification of topics and speakers. This workshop summary was prepared by the rapporteurs as a factual summary of the presentations and discussions that took place at the workshop. Statements, recommendations, and opinions expressed are those of the individual presenters and participants, are not necessarily endorsed or verified by the IOM or the National Cancer Policy Forum, and should not be construed as reflecting any group consensus.

OVERVIEW OF KEY POINTS HIGHLIGHTED BY INDIVIDUAL PRESENTERS

Cancer researchers and care providers are facing an overwhelming volume of data from a multitude of sources and are hampered by the inability to merge those data or to communicate effectively across disciplines and stakeholders because of divergent standards, lack of interoperability, and other barriers.

Biomedical informatics could be advanced by

- abandoning siloed datasets for large-scale, standardized, interoperable open source databases with professional annotation, analytics, and curation;
- integrating research and clinical data in an organized and efficient manner;
- supporting an open source platform for the development of software; and
- considering secondary uses of IT infrastructure as a way to reduce overall costs.

The clinical translational research process could be advanced by

- bringing routinely gathered clinical data up to the same standards as high-quality research data;
- developing new statistical methods and study designs for use with clinical data;
- developing better data mining and filtering approaches to sort through massive datasets;
- connecting genomic and molecular data with clinical data;
- structuring clinical data appropriately to support research;
- integrating data that are already in the public domain to generate new hypotheses for testing;
- ensuring that these processes are guided in a way that is compatible with a research framework; and
- using a systems view of disease, which postulates that disease is the result of perturbation of one or more biological networks that leads to altered expression of information, to address the complexity of biology.

continued

> Clinical cancer care could be improved by
>
> - developing frameworks that can help clinicians make progressively better care decisions with each individual patient, even in the absence of gold standard data;
> - making it easier for every oncology practice to care for a patient on a clinical trial protocol; and
> - developing a coalition as a nonprofit membership organization comprised of all stakeholders, who are deeply committed to actualizing a common vision of data liquidity to achieve personalized cancer care and a rapid-learning health care system.
>
> Patient engagement could be enhanced by
>
> - building trust through improved transparency, both to the public at large and to patients, about how patient data are used, the typical tools that institutions use to protect data, and oversight and accountability for those protections;
> - empowering patients to drive disruptive innovation in health care; and
> - providing more guidance about how to comply with the Health Insurance Portability and Accountability Act (HIPAA) Privacy Rule.

ORGANIZATION OF THE WORKSHOP AND SUMMARY

The report that follows summarizes the presentations and discussions by the expert panelists and participants. As introduced by Sharon Murphy, scholar-in-residence at the IOM, the workshop was organized into three main panel sessions. The first panel session provided an overview of the informatics landscape and framed the issues from a variety of stakeholder perspectives, including clinical and translational research, epidemiology and biostatistics, major cancer centers, and cancer cooperative groups (Chapter 2). Following the overview, the keynote address was delivered by Leroy Hood of the Institute for Systems Biology, focusing on the role of informatics in personalized medicine (Chapter 3). The second panel session incorporated several illustrative "use cases" reflecting successful informatics-supported approaches to managing large, complex datasets, including data collection, storage, and retrieval; data analysis and reporting; and data sharing (Chapter 4). The third panel session challenged participants to look forward and consider new models and potential strategies to advance informatics as a community and reap the most value from the huge investment in cancer research (Chapter 5). A proposal for a broad stakeholder coalition as one pathway for addressing the informatics needs of the cancer research community was also described (Chapter 6). In closing the workshop, Amy Abernethy, associate professor of medicine in the Division of Medical Oncology at the Duke University School of Medicine, offered reflections on the themes discussed and summarized the suggestions made for moving forward (Chapter 7).

REFERENCES

IOM (Institute of Medicine). 2010. *A foundation for evidence-driven practice: A rapid learning system for cancer care: Workshop summary.* Washington, DC: The National Academies Press.

IOM. 2011. *Digital infrastructure for the learning health system: The foundation for continuous improvement in health and health care: Workshop series summary.* Washington, DC: The National Academies Press.

Miriovsky, B. J., L. N. Shulman, and A. P. Abernethy. 2012. In press. Importance of health information technology, electronic health records and continuously aggregating data to comparative effectiveness research and learning health care. *Journal of Clinical Oncology.*

2

Overview of the Cancer Informatics Landscape

> **DISCUSSION POINTS HIGHLIGHTED BY INDIVIDUAL PRESENTERS**
>
> - Cancer researchers and care providers are facing an overwhelming volume of data from a multitude of sources and are hampered by the inability to merge those data or to communicate effectively across disciplines and stakeholders because of divergent standards, lack of interoperability, and other barriers.
> - The most successful informatics tools will be those that integrate research and clinical data in an organized and efficient manner.
> - A research information exchange system integrates data from multiple sources (extracting, transforming, harmonizing, and profiling for quality and accuracy) and then makes them available to diverse stakeholders per their queries. The information is provided based on the same data elements, but the presentation depends on who is asking for it (researchers, patients, clinicians, or administrators).
> - Guiding principles for an integrated data warehouse include relevant standards for data entry, deep annotation, a good query interface, and sharing (via entry back into the database) of any new data derived from the analysis of data, specimens, or images stored in the data warehouse.
>
> *continued*

- Research data sources span the spectrum from electronic health records (EHRs) to disease registries to clinical research protocol repositories, with varying degrees of completeness, quality, and research utility. In silico research depends on having complete and valid information.
- caBIG is undergoing renovations and new informatics project review criteria are being implemented; NCI is open and receptive to communications from interested parties.

In the first session, an overview of the current status of cancer informatics was provided from the perspectives of cancer centers, cancer cooperative groups, and clinical translational researchers. Panelists also discussed the lessons that could be learned from the ongoing evolution of NCI's caBIG.

STRUCTURED, INTEROPERABLE RESEARCH AND CLINICAL INFORMATION SYSTEMS—OR THE LACK THEREOF

Data Overload

Rapid advances in technology have led to a dramatic increase in the output of genomic and molecular data related to cancer biology, said Lawrence Shulman, chief medical officer and chief of the Division of General Oncology at the Dana-Farber Cancer Institute. These emerging data can inform our understanding of basic cancer biology, epidemiology, and behavior, as well as response to therapies, toxicity of therapies, and optimal care for an individual patient or cohort. However, the sheer volume of information presents significant data management and analysis challenges and is becoming overwhelming from a clinical decision-making standpoint.

To be optimally useful, data should be structured in a database, and we are still in the learning stages of how best to structure genomic and molecular data, Shulman noted. For clinical data to be useful, they should contain certain critical elements. From an oncology perspective, examples of key data elements include patient demographics; tumor type and anatomic and non-anatomic staging; treatment plan, treatment intent (e.g., curative or palliative), and actual treatment; tumor response; toxicity; patient-reported outcomes; and disease-free and overall survival. The nation is moving, albeit slowly, toward the adoption of electronic health records (EHRs) to facilitate efficient clinical practice and decision making. However, many of the data included in EHRs are not in a structured format (i.e., are entered as free text). One must often read through the notes of clinicians, and it can be challenging to discern exactly what has happened to the patient, Shulman said.

Databases That Foster Learning

Shulman stressed that the most successful informatics tools will be those that interconnect research, clinical activities, and data in an organized and efficient manner, with as broad a database as possible. Citing a 2010 IOM workshop on evidence-driven practice in cancer care, he explained that the patient is the center of the system around which there is a cycle of aggregating information (including routinely collected real-time clinical data), analyzing that information, making new discoveries, and applying those discoveries to improve the care of individual patients (Abernethy et al., 2010; IOM, 2010) (Figure 2-1). The American Society of Clinical Oncology has recently launched CancerLinQ,[1] a rapid-learning system based on this model that is being pilot-tested first for breast cancer. Shulman described an example in place at Dana-Farber, called the Synergistic Patient and Research Knowledge Systems (SPARKS) (Box 2-1; Figure 2-2). This system links clinical data (e.g., EHR, surgical, and pathology data), tissue sample information, cancer registry information, patient-reported outcomes, translational research data (e.g., gene expression), and operations data (e.g., billing, scheduling, and other visit information).

Making Connections

Shulman offered the "life cycle" of a gene mutation as a practical example of the value of an integrated data system. In this scenario, a basic researcher discovers a gene mutation in the laboratory, but its clinical significance is unclear. An association with a clinical syndrome is then determined. Translational research ties that gene mutation to a clinical outcome (e.g., prognosis, response to therapy). The clinical significance of the mutation is validated, and testing for the mutation may have therapeutic implications.

---

[1] See http://www.asco.org/ASCOv2/Practice+%26+Guidelines/Quality+Care/CancerLinQ+-+Building+a+Transformation+in+Cancer+Care.

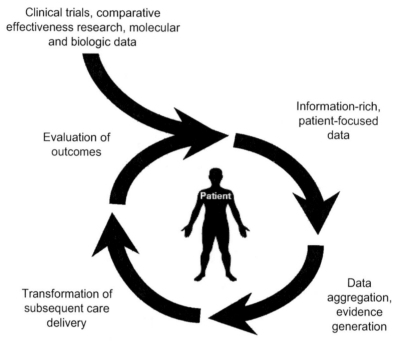

FIGURE 2-1 Rapid-learning health care system for cancer care.
SOURCE: Abernethy et al., 2010; IOM, 2010.

At Dana-Farber, researchers can query both a clinical data repository and a consented research database. A "transient data mart" houses data involved in a current query, which is then purged when the query is completed. Data are de-identified, and queries are covered under an umbrella protocol so that additional institutional review board (IRB) approval is not required. Investigators could be seeking an actionable mutation in multiple tumor types and could query, for example, the aggregate number of patients who have human epidermal growth factor receptor 2 (HER2) amplification in breast, gastric, and salivary gland tumors and have responded to trastuzumab. Queries can be very specific. For example, an investigator interested in hormone resistance might query the frequency of a particular mutation in women who have metastatic breast cancer that is estrogen receptor (ER)-positive and HER2-positive, who are between the ages of 50 and 65, and who had progressive disease while on tamoxifen. It is also possible to access identified data with IRB approval, and investigators recruiting for a

> **BOX 2-1**
> **Dana-Farber Synergistic Patient and Research Knowledge Systems (SPARKS)**
>
> **Vision** To provide a cutting-edge, collaborative institutional informatics framework to accelerate scientific discoveries and their translation into clinical practice to enable early diagnosis, personalized treatment, cure, and prevention of cancer and related diseases.
>
> **Objective** Implement policies, standards, systems, and tools that facilitate collection, integration, mining, analysis, and interpretation of biomedical data to accelerate scientific discoveries and their translation into personalized medicine and clinical practice.
>
> **Long-term goal** Establish an integrated, patient-centric clinical genomic data model and systems for enabling translational research and personalized medicine.
>
> NOTE: See also Figure 2-2.
> SOURCE: Shulman presentation (February 27, 2012).

particular investigational protocol could query for actual patients who meet specific eligibility criteria.

Robust EHR Systems and Research Databases

In closing, Shulman stressed the need for robust EHR systems and robust research databases. All clinical data in EHRs should be codified or structured, he said. EHRs should include detailed data on patient demographics, tumor characteristics and staging, and treatment histories, as well as codified treatment responses and treatment resistance development and codified genomic and molecular data. Ideally, EHR systems would be interoperable and have standards for data entry. Similarly, he said there is need for robust, interoperable research databases containing structured genomic and molecular data, entered according to defined standards, and these research databases should link with relevant clinical databases. Shulman said that we are not even close to these aspirations.

Such databases often exist at the laboratory level and, in many cases,

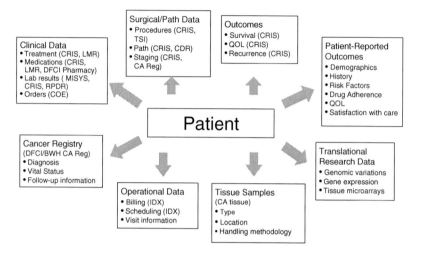

FIGURE 2-2 Dana-Farber Synergistic Patient and Research Knowledge Systems (SPARKS).
NOTE: BWH = Brigham and Women's Cancer Center; CA = cancer; CDR = Clinical Data Repository; COE = computer order entry for chemotherapy and all medications; CRIS = Clinical Research Information System; DFCI = Dana-Farber Cancer Institute; IDX = IDX operating system; LMR = longitudinal electronic medical record; Path = pathological; QOL = quality of life; Reg = registry; RPDR = Research Patient Data Registry.
SOURCE: Shulman presentation (February 27, 2012).

at the institutional (e.g., cancer center) level. To be maximally effective, however, Shulman said, there is a need for database efforts at a national or even international level, incorporating data from academic centers as well as community practices (where about 80 percent of patients in the United States receive their cancer care).

CANCER CENTER INFORMATICS: CONNECTING WITH PATIENTS

To integrate new technologies into the standard of care there must be demonstrated value, explained William Dalton, president, CEO, and center director of the H. Lee Moffitt Cancer Center & Research Institute.[2] A given treatment or technology, however, may not provide the same value

---

[2] In July 2012, Dr. Dalton assumed the position of CEO for the newly formed M2Gen Personalized Medicine Institute at the Moffitt Cancer Center.

to all patients. Evidence must be generated regarding what works for which individuals or cohorts. Dalton outlined four elements of a personalized medicine approach that can lead to overall improved health care:

1. Addresses health care as a public issue and seeks to *improve access, affordability, and quality of care* by developing an information system to assist in making clinical decisions based on outcomes and comparative effectiveness;
2. *Integrates new technologies* into the standard of care *in an evidence-based fashion* to identify populations at risk, personalize treatment, and improve individual outcomes;
3. Provides an approach to identify the *best treatment for individual patients* based on clinical and biological characteristics of patients and their disease; and
4. Creates a *network of health care providers, patients, and researchers* who contribute and share information from individual patients to ultimately improve the care of all patients by learning from the experience of others (Dalton et al., 2010).

Research Information Exchange

Improved medical care begins with data that provide information, from which we derive knowledge and develop wisdom, and we are still in the data phase of this journey, Dalton said. In implementing a research information exchange system that will serve the key stakeholders, cancers centers face technical, cultural (e.g., academic versus industry), regulatory, and financial challenges. From a technical and regulatory standpoint, data sharing raises many issues that must be addressed, for example, technical architecture, intellectual property concerns, privacy and security, and human subjects' protections.

Another, perhaps underappreciated, technical aspect is data governance, Dalton said. How are the validity and quality of the data entered into the system ensured? Semantic interoperability or harmonization is needed; the system must serve users who are looking for the same data but in a different context or with different semantics and syntax, depending on who is asking. Multiple data sources can actually help ensure data quality, Dalton suggested.

The challenge is how to develop an integrated network information system that can manage the ever-increasing amount of information being generated in basic, translational, and clinical research that is needed to support a personalized medicine approach. Dalton pointed out that a single information system can serve multiple stakeholders, including researchers, patients, administrators, and clinicians. Information is provided based on the same data or "truth," but the presentation will depend on who is asking for it. As noted by Shulman, a database can be used by researchers to identify a patient cohort for data analysis or for clinical trial recruitment. Researchers might also seek data on comparative effectiveness or to do molecular profiling. The same information system, Dalton said, should allow patients to have their own personalized health record, which they can interact with and contribute to. The same platform would also be able to support evidence-based decision making by clinicians and administrators.

Dalton offered an illustration showing how an information exchange system could be designed (Figure 2-3). The goal was to develop a system

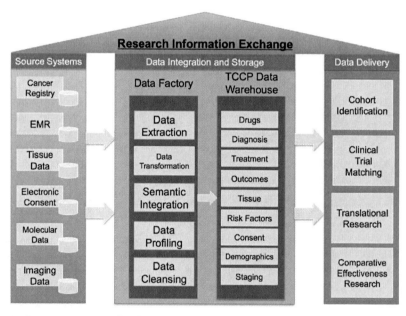

FIGURE 2-3 Example of a research information exchange system at the Moffitt Cancer Center, integrating data from multiple sources and providing them to diverse stakeholders.
NOTE: EMR = electronic medical record; TCCP = Total Cancer Care Protocol.
SOURCE: Fenstermacher et al., 2011. Reprinted with permission from *The Cancer Journal.*

that could identify the same patient in multiple source data systems that may use different identification numbers or ways of describing the patient. The data are loaded into a "data factory" where they are extracted, transformed, harmonized, and profiled for quality and accuracy. Data are then stored in the warehouse to be delivered to stakeholders per their queries. In response to a question about the broad integrity of the informatics enterprise, Dalton stressed the emphasis that the data factory places on ensuring the quality of data before they enter the data warehouse. In addition, multiple sources of data on the same individual allow for algorithm checks for quality.

It was noted by a participant that a challenge in obtaining patient consent for inclusion in such systems is ensuring that patients understand what they are consenting to, specifically that their data may be used for studies that are not yet defined to answer questions that have not yet been thought of. A multiphased consent process, where patients can opt in or opt out of different parts of the program, may be most appropriate, but it is a complicated and lengthy process. Dalton shared the example of a large, ongoing observational study in which patients consented to be studied throughout their lifetime, including collecting tumor samples and being recontacted should the investigators find something that might benefit them. An analysis of patient comprehension found that over time, many had forgotten that they had consented to this ongoing interaction. To help address this, patients receive a card within 2 weeks of consenting that thanks them for enrolling in the study, including a phone number to call if they have questions or do not recall consenting. A patient portal has also been developed, Dalton said, which again thanks patients for consenting and explains that they can obtain information about how their data are being used and how they can opt out at any time.

CANCER COOPERATIVE GROUP INFORMATICS: CONNECTING RESEARCHERS

Robert Comis, president and chair of the Coalition of Cancer Cooperative Groups and group chair of the Eastern Cooperative Oncology Group (ECOG), provided an overview of the NCI Clinical Trials Cooperative Group Program. As a result of an ongoing reconfiguration of the cooperative group structure, the program now comprises five major groups:

1. **Alliance for Clinical Trials in Oncology**—merging the Cancer and Leukemia Group B (CALGB), the North Central Cancer Treatment

Group (NCCTG), and the American College of Surgeons Oncology Group (ACOSOG);
2. **Children's Oncology Group;**
3. **ECOG-ACRIN Cancer Research Group**—merging the American College of Radiology Imaging Network (ACRIN) and ECOG;
4. **NRG Oncology Group**—merging the National Surgical Adjuvant Breast and Bowel Project (NSABP), the Radiation Therapy Oncology Group (RTOG), and the Gynecologic Oncology Group; and
5. **SWOG** (formerly the Southwest Oncology Group).

Comis explained that the cooperative group environment includes academic centers, large community practices, smaller community practices, and biomedical researchers spanning the physical sciences through the clinical sciences. It is geographically dispersed and now includes international sites.

Historically, cooperative group clinical trial results have been crucial to setting the standards of cancer care. The primary mode of data collection has been case report forms, which are stored in individual group databases. There are some ad hoc interfaces for reporting and local information technology systems for managing tissue samples.

In 1999, NCI established the Cancer Trials Support Unit (CTSU), which, Comis said, now serves around 1,700 sites and thousands of investigators, supporting patient enrollment and randomization, data collection using common data elements, and regulatory and administrative activities.

Informatics Tools Used by the NCI Cooperative Group Program

Comis described the development and implementation of the Medidata Rave Clinical Data Management System software now used by the Cooperative Group Program. In 2005, the cooperative groups recognized that there was a need for a unified data system across the program. Specifications were developed; a request for proposals was sent to several vendors; and in 2008, a contract was awarded to Medidata. The unsuccessful vendors then filed formal protests, stalling the start of the contracted work. Following resolution of the disputes, the program was officially initiated in April 2011, resulting in Rave, a web-based system for capturing, managing, and reporting clinical research data that enables the user to record patient information using forms customized per study (visit, lab, and adverse event data). The program is now managed by the NCI Cancer Therapy and Evaluation Program (CTEP), with the assistance of the CTSU and Medidata, and involves all of the cooperative groups. Hundreds of group representatives are currently engaged in classroom, webinar, and e-learning training on how to use the Rave system.

Another effort Comis described focuses on coordinating the tissue banking activities across cooperative groups. The Group Banking Committee, sponsored by NCI, is developing processes and standards for a national groupwide tissue bank virtual repository. Comis noted that each tissue bank has developed its own biospecimen information management system. Some systems integrate multiple banks, and some systems are integrated with institutional information technology (IT) systems. In addition, some groups have specimen tracking systems, which connect data entry at clinical sites with trial operations systems and bank inventory systems. The goal is to connect the various group IT structures to a single database that can be queried and is available to all researchers throughout the country.

Opportunities for an Innovative Informatics Structure

Mitchell Schnall, group chair of ACRIN, described some of the opportunities for cooperative groups in building an innovative informatics structure. Cooperative groups are a rich source of diverse biosamples and images that are associated with structured clinical information, often with long-term follow-up. In addition, there is a large array of other information, ranging from gross medical and histological images to molecular data profiling genes and proteins, that needs to be integrated with the clinical information.

The ECOG-ACRIN vision, Schnall explained, is to generate an integrated data warehouse incorporating the individual case report form, such as that from the Medidata Rave system, with imaging data, laboratory data, tissue and specimen repository inventory, digitized pathology, and -omics data (e.g., genomics, metabolomics, proteomics) as well as patient-reported outcomes and claims data.

Schnall offered several guiding principles for moving forward with such a system. First, it will be necessary for the cooperative groups to embrace relevant standards. Deep annotation should be encouraged (e.g., spatial annotation), a good query interface is important, and any new data that are derived from analysis of ECOG-ACRIN specimens or images should be entered into the data warehouse to further the value of the warehouse as a community resource. With regard to deep annotation, Schnall said that cancer control moves along a pathway from prevention to detection and characterization and then through treatment, response assessment, adaptation of therapy, and surveillance. We need to understand the data in terms of where they were derived along this disease pathway. In addition, data can be structured relative to patient level, disease level, lesion level, and even sublesion level.

One of the tools ACRIN could contribute to an integrated data warehouse, for example, is TRIAD, a standards-based server and database that was developed to facilitate the exchange of imaging data. Currently in use at more than 200 sites, TRIAD is compliant with Good Clinical Practice (GCP) and houses image data from more than 100,000 cases, which are integrated with clinical data from the Medidata Rave system.

One concern with current image repositories, Schnall noted, is that information defining a specific location on the image is not retained after the analysis is finished. There is variability within a single tumor or among multiple lesions in a single patient, and such specificity is needed to be able to track lesions over time and over modalities and to tie pathology data directly to a specific lesion. A standard that ACRIN is embracing is called Annotation and Image Markup (AIM), which allows reviewers to set up a region of interest in an image for which they can add metadata describing that region of interest. This is very valuable for indexing specific lesions, Schnall said. Another goal is to be able to link a specific pathological or histological section with the location in the anatomic image that it came from. This goes beyond simply saying that a particular bit of data came from a patient that had breast cancer, to knowing what part of the histological specimen the molecular data came from and what specific part of the tumor the pathology sample came from.

The ECOG-ACRIN goal for the future is to have a central operations "cloud" linked to the administration and operations functions and the data sources. Interested stakeholder communities (e.g., clinical sites, the scientific community, scientific programs, patients, NCI) would then be able to interface with that cloud.

CLINICAL TRANSLATIONAL RESEARCH INFORMATICS: CONNECTING THE STEPS OF THE RESEARCH PROCESS

Bradley Pollock is chair of the Department of Epidemiology and Biostatistics at the University of Texas Health Science Center at San Antonio. He is also chair-elect of the Biostatistics, Epidemiology, and Research Design Committee of a national consortium funded by NIH through a Clinical & Translational Science Award (CTSA). He outlined the steps in the research process for clinical translational studies as follows: hypothesis formation, study design and planning, data acquisition, statistical modeling and analysis, drawing valid inferences, and translation. While data are the critical basic building blocks, the development of evidence-based practice guidelines is driven by the entire research process.

Hypothesis Driven Versus Hypothesis Generating

Traditionally, the first step of the research process is to develop the hypothesis for which one will then design an experiment and collect data. Now, research is experiencing a paradigm shift as a result of the ever-increasing generation and availability of observational data Pollock said. We now have data, but remain in search of hypotheses. While hypothesis-generating work is important, he noted that the most novel oncology discoveries have been made using the traditional hypothesis-driven research framework.

Study Design

In clinical research, attention to study design is extremely important. Good design leads to efficient use of data, and study design can have profound implications for validity. As a testament to the importance of study design for obtaining meaningful results, Pollock noted that the *New England Journal of Medicine* now requests full protocols for all clinical trials.

The randomized, controlled trial (RCT) is the gold standard for clinical studies; however, an RCT is not applicable or feasible in all situations. In designing observational studies, Pollock suggested that there may be more methodological hurdles to overcome than for RCTs. He cited a recent report of how the inclusion of incident versus prevalent cases in an observational study of postmenopausal hormone replacement therapy affected the results (Danaei et al., 2012). There have been concerns about the discordance between randomized versus observational studies of the effects of hormone replacement therapy on cardiovascular disease in women. In their meta-analysis, the researchers found that exclusion of prevalent users of hormone replacement therapy decreased the discrepancies between observational and randomized studies. Pollock questioned whether nuances such as prevalent versus incident use could reliably be discerned from EHRs when conducting observational studies.

In designing a research study, one generally begins by combing the literature. Unfortunately, the value of the literature for informing study design is negatively affected by publication bias and the lag time between study findings and their final publication. The trial registry, ClinicalTrials.gov, is a useful resource but is limited to clinical trials, and entries do not provide a level of detail, rigor, or standardization necessary for scientific analysis. There is a real need, Pollock said, for accessible meta-study data for all types of study designs (not just clinical trials).

In this regard, Pollock drew attention to the Human Studies Database Project, a database of past and ongoing human studies, both interventional and observational. The primary project participants are CTSA institutions. Pollock said that the goal is to enable computational reuse of human studies data for activities such as systematic reviews, planning future studies, scientific portfolio analysis, and research networking. A subcomponent of the project is the Ontology of Clinical Research (OCRe), focused on developing an ontology to deal with issues of study design, interventions and exposures, participants, outcomes, and statistical analysis.

Informatics Challenges for Translational Research

Studies Using Existing, Non-Research Data

Research data sources span the spectrum from EHRs to disease registries to clinical research protocol repositories, with varying degrees of completeness, quality, and research utility. Pollock concurred with Shulman regarding the need for structured data elements. In EHRs, for example, useful information about drug exposure would include dose, schedule, intensity, area under the curve, dose modifications, reasons for stopping a drug, and patient pharmacokinetics, pharmacodynamics, and pharmacogenomic characteristics. These data are not generally included in the EHR, however. The major challenge when using existing information, Pollock said, is the inability to go back and fill in the missing data needed for a particular research investigation. Another concern with mining existing data is the potential for systematic biases in large clinical data repositories. More data is not necessarily better, Pollock noted, and biases can be amplified. In silico research depends on having complete and valid information.

Lack of Harmonization

From the perspective of a clinical translational researcher, Pollock concurred with the challenges highlighted by the cancer centers and cooperative groups. Lack of harmonization is a key concern, and he noted that at his own institution, as in many academic health centers, there is more than one EHR system in place. Clinical data systems and research data systems do not routinely interoperate. Another issue for clinical research is the choice of clinical trial management system (CTMS) and whether to use a commercially available system or an open source system. There are sustainability and cost issues to consider. Open source is technically free, but not without cost because a lot more development time goes into implementing an open source platform; however, it may be more sustainable when moving forward.

Regulatory Barriers

There are also regulatory barriers for public use datasets. As chair of the advisory committee for the Texas Cancer Registry, Pollock expressed concerns about the heterogeneity of across-state permissions to combine data from multiple state cancer registries (in some cases, four levels of approval are required before researchers can utilize the data). There are also within-state restrictions; for example, until very recently, linking hospital discharge data and Texas Cancer Registry data was not permitted.

Tools, Technology, and Big Datasets

Imaging data are highly dimensional, and technical advances, such as the ability to collect real-time functional imaging data, further increase data dimensionality. There also has been an explosion in -omics data and analysis tools. Decision support tools are available, but they require large-scale validation and constant updating. Limitations to data storage and networking are also a major issue. In one genome sequencing laboratory Pollock had visited, for example, it was possible to keep active datasets on the server for only about 1 week, after which the data had to be pulled off to create space for new data.

Despite the challenges, big datasets can facilitate hypothesis generation and study planning. Data can be used to assess the feasibility of a study. Big datasets could also lower the cost of conducting clinical translational research, Pollock said, by offering more precollected data, more automation, and more interconnectivity.

Moving Clinical Translational Informatics Forward

Pollock reiterated that research is a process, and more data do not necessarily lead to more discovery. He offered several suggestions to help evolve the clinical translational research process:

- Bring clinical data up to the same standards as high-quality research data.
- Devise statistical methodologies and study designs for use with clinical data.
- Develop better data mining and filtering approaches to sort through massive datasets.
- Connect genomic and molecular data with clinical data.
- Structure clinical data appropriately to support research.
- Ensure that these processes are guided in a way that is compatible with a research framework.

caBIG—THE VISION AND THE REALITY

Daniel Masys, affiliate professor of biomedical and health informatics at the University of Washington, Seattle, and chair of the new caBIG oversight subcommittee of the NCI Board of Scientific Advisors, shared the history and vision of caBIG and some of the lessons learned since its launch in 2004. The Cancer Biomedical Informatics Grid was launched by NCI to help address the growing problem of the overwhelming volume of data from a multitude of sources and the inability to merge those data or to communicate effectively across disciplines and stakeholders because of divergent standards and terms and other barriers.

To define the priority areas for caBIG, a very extensive market determination exercise was undertaken to define the unmet needs of the NCI-supported cancer centers (Box 2-2). As a result, caBIG was envisioned as a common, widely distributed infrastructure that would permit the research community to focus on innovation (rather than on the details of managing information), with the intent that raw and published cancer research data would be available for data mining and integration into reanalyses and meta-analyses. It would be built on shared vocabulary, data elements, and data models that would facilitate information exchange and would have a collection of interoperable applications and tools developed with common standards.

> **BOX 2-2**
> **Common Needs to Catalyze Effectiveness in Cancer Research That Helped to Shape the Priority Areas for the caBIG Activities**
>
> - Clinical data management tools
> - Distributed data sharing/analysis tools
> - Translational research tools
> - Access to data
> - Tissue and pathology tools
> - Cancer center integration and program management
> - Common data elements and standards
> - Meta-data analysis
> - Shared vocabulary and ontology tools and databases
> - Statistical data analysis tools
> - Visualization and imaging tools
> - Proteomics
> - Microarray and gene expression tools
> - Licensing and intellectual property issues
> - Staff resources
> - High-performance computing
> - Integration and interoperability
>
> SOURCE: Masys presentation (February 27, 2012).

In 2010, NCI director Harold Varmus called for a high-level review of caBIG. In its report released in March 2011, the working group concluded that the need for caBIG is greater now then when it was conceived (NCI, 2011). In addition, there was very strong community support from cancer centers for the original caBIG vision and goals of interoperability and standards-based exchange of data. The working group also found, however, that the many successes of the program have been offset by several problems and that the overall impact of caBIG in transforming cancer research had not been commensurate with the level of the investment (about $300 million).

The report highlighted findings in three main areas:

1. creation and management of standards for data exchange, and support for community-based software already in place;

2. impact and track record of caBIG initiatives and tools with regard to life science or integrative cancer research, clinical data management, infrastructure, and community engagement; and
3. program administration, contracts management, and budget.

The working group concluded that the greatest impact of caBIG thus far had been in the first area. The review found that the program had been very effective in catalyzing progress in the development of community-driven standards for data exchange and interoperability; development, maintenance, enhancement, and dissemination of tools developed by academic researchers; and community dialogue on the interoperability of clinical and research software tools.

The group found that the main problems with the caBIG approach that limited its uptake and impact included a "cart-before-the-horse grand vision"; a technology-centric approach to data sharing; unfocused expansion; a one-size-fits-all architectural approach; an unsustainable business model for both NCI and users; and a lack of independent scientific oversight.

As a result, the working group issued five immediate tactical recommendations. They are, as summarized by Masys:

1. Institute an immediate moratorium on all ongoing internal and commercial contractor-based software development projects while initiating a mitigation plan to lessen the impact of this moratorium on the cancer research community.
2. Institute a 1-year moratorium on new projects, contracts, and subcontracts by caBIG.
3. Provide a 1-year extension on current caBIG-supported academic efforts for development, dissemination, and maintenance of new and existing community-developed software tools.
4. Establish an independent oversight committee, representing academic, industrial, and government (NCI, National Institutes of Health [NIH]) perspectives to review planned initiatives for scientific merit and to recommend effective transition options for current users of caBIG tools.
5. Conduct a thorough audit of all aspects of the caBIG budget and expenditures.

The independent oversight committee that was called for in recommendation 4 (chaired by Masys) met for first time in July 2011. To begin to address the criticisms in the March report, the committee developed review criteria for informatics projects (similar to the evaluation criteria used by study sections), outlining how it would assess each of the ongoing caBIG activities, Masys noted (Box 2-3).

Looking Forward: A Three-Step Approach to Success in Informatics Innovation

In response to a request from the NCI director, Masys consulted with other experts to try to define the "recipe for success," that is, are there comparable programs that have been successful and what can we learn from them? Masys found that two applications had "gone viral": the Research Electronic Data Capture (REDCap) developed through a CTSA, and the Informatics for Integrating Biology and the Bedside (i2b2), developed with funding from NIH's National Center for Biomedical Computing. In considering how these applications were different from caBIG, Masys and colleagues drafted the following general steps to success in informatics innovation.

1. **Do not repeat the mistakes of the past.**
   - Do not try to solve all clinical and translational research information technology problems in one framework.
   - Do not worship standards over functionality.
   - Do not try to have enterprise software adopted by fiat from above.
   - Do not try to buy adoption software products, because for the sponsor, those costs grow ever larger.
   - Recognize that organizations that cannot afford ongoing staffing and help desk functions for software should not be expected to adopt software even if it is free or provides some income to the adopter. The acquisition cost is dwarfed by the support, maintenance, and integration costs.

2. **Understand the basic truth about IT complexity.**
Increased functionality that is built at the expense of increased complexity is always at risk of
   - delays in development,
   - inability of local implementers and users to understand what has been built and how to use it, and
   - being overtaken by other approaches that have a better price-to-performance ratio (e.g., grid computing versus web services).

BOX 2-3
NCI Informatics Project Review Criteria

1. Does the activity, application, or resource meet a well-articulated and attainable need of basic, translational, or clinical research, or cancer care (i.e., is there a "driving biological or clinical project" and are the intended users members of the project team)?
2. How will success or failure be evaluated? Analogous to stopping rules for clinical protocols, what will be the stopping rules for ending the project if it either fails to meet its technical objectives or fails to be adopted even if technically successful?
3. Will the activity, resource, or application, if successful, make some objectively measurable incremental progress toward an overall vision of interoperability of data and systems? Will it enable data sharing and make use of and/or enhance open international standards for research?
4. Is the activity, resource, or application designed to anticipate change in a rapidly expanding knowledge base of science and practice? Flexibility and generalizability are important characteristics for longevity in an era of agile science.
5. Is the intended deliverable of the project achievable in the time frame and budget proposed?
6. Will the output of the project be broadly implementable by organizations of varying size and sophistication? Will it be used broadly by organizations and institutions outside of NCI cancer centers (e.g., other NIH centers or academic research organizations)?
7. Is there a documented plan for long-term maintenance, enhancement, and fiscal sustainability of the activity, application, or resource and its user base?
8. What is the user base and has there been a stakeholder assessment to ensure that the activity, application, or resource will indeed meet a currently unmet need or a reasonably anticipated future need?
9. Is the project generalizable and likely to create value or address broad needs across the community of cancer centers and investigators? Alternatively, would this activity, resource, or application be perceived as a "pet project" of an "in" group?
10. Does the activity, resource, or application have enough market value to gain adoption without incentives? Or if financial or policy incentives are required, are they justified?

SOURCE: Masys presentation (February 27, 2012).

3. Observe the informatics research and development "do's."
- Solve one significant challenge at a time.
- Use small, nimble development teams led by domain experts.
- Keep development-to-implementation intervals short.
- Deploy software that can solve at least one problem that users or adopters care about within 12 months of adoption.
- Demonstrate success first with a smaller group of the most advanced sites and then let others follow.
- Create software that makes adoption of standards easier (not harder) than nonstandardized alternatives.
- Let the market prioritize and vet the standards.
- Invest in simple interfaces between applications, not architectures.
- Make interested health care organizations demonstrate willingness to invest their own assets and time for enterprise software.
- Allow intraorganizational and interorganizational needs and technologies to diverge as needed, to maximize productivity.

With regard to increasing the probability of successful adoption of informatics innovation in cancer research specifically, Masys recommended focusing data sharing efforts (both the standards for sharing and the applications to do it) on those data for which there is a preexisting motivation to share. Areas in which researchers really need one another's data and scientific problems that simply cannot be solved within one laboratory or institution are prime areas on which to focus sharing efforts (e.g., those studying rare alleles who are trying to assemble a cohort of interest for a study). Cooperative groups are a good example of this, he noted. The current challenges are less technological and more policy oriented (e.g., IRB issues, privacy concerns).

Increasing the uptake of innovative informatics in cancer care is a more difficult task, given the low penetrance of EHRs in U.S. health care and current economic pressures. Therefore, Masys advised aligning NCI efforts with the EHR adoption incentives of the Office of the National Coordinator for Health Information Technology (discussed further by Mostashari in Chapter 5). A plausible transition goal for NCI, he suggested, would be to make it easier for every oncology practice in America to care for a patient on a clinical trial protocol. Building "public libraries" of decision support tools to guide providers and patients through clinical protocols would be an important contribution in this regard.

Community Participation in Moving Informatics Forward

During the discussion, there was much interest in involving patients as well as the research community in efforts to advance cancer informatics. Questions remain regarding how best to interact with NCI on caBIG activities, the potential role of publicly developed apps, open source software, the development of institutional systems, and the importance of patient-reported outcomes data.

NCI is very open and receptive to communications from interested parties, Masys said. George Komatsoulis, interim director for the Center for Biomedical Informatics and Information Technology at NCI, added that caBIG is continuing to move forward, and there are "workspaces" in integrative basic biology, clinical trials, data standards, imaging, biospecimens, and other areas where individuals can bring their ideas to the attention of the scientific advisory group and the caBIG program staff.

Lynn Etheredge of George Washington University asked if a national apps strategy for cancer informatics would be appropriate, that is, whether individuals could begin to develop the needed functionalities. Masys noted that apps, as they are commonly understood, tend to be fairly small-scale computer programs. They have value as lightweight applications that handle very common tasks on a personal level, often on a personal device such as a smartphone or tablet. However, their level of complexity is usually around two orders of magnitude less than enterprise-level software (e.g., that used by researchers for regular data inputs required for supporting sponsors), with lower levels of data manipulation, storage, and security. Enterprise-level software requires a more in-depth approach to implementation and, in health care and clinical research, may also involve workflow modification.

Steven Piantadosi asked about open source software relative to caBIG. Masys responded that open source software is part of the caBIG infrastructure: i2b2 is open source, while REDCap is an academic consortium model where a limited number of people have the ability to contribute to the code base. Masys cautioned that in a full open source software model (where anybody in the community can contribute to source), modules can be introduced that have unintended transitive consequences (i.e., interfere with other functions). As such, some open source models use quality control mechanisms such as curators or stewards.

Mendelsohn noted that many organizations are trying to develop their own internal standardized record of clinical trials and asked whether these organizations should continue to spend scarce resources, time, and effort developing these independent information systems in light of the national effort.

Masys responded that any major cancer center is going to have two overlapping spheres of development, one that is outwardly focused and one that is local and specific to the organization. There will then be transition applications that facilitate sharing sets of data by formatting them and ensuring that they meet the standard for external collaborations. The cooperative groups, for example, are well served by tools such as Medidata Rave, which, while not perfect, is implemented on a large scale and provides a conceptual basis for sharing information, he said.

Mark Gorman, cancer survivor and patient advocate, expressed support for the patient-centered elements of the information systems discussed, for example, those designed to collect patient-reported outcome information. There is also great potential for informatics to support patients in their decision making and in managing their own care. Dalton noted that patient portals are very popular, with more than 70 percent of new cancer patients at Moffitt creating their portal before their first visit. Shulman added that the power of the systems discussed is the multiple sources of complementary data obtained by different methodologies, and this includes the patient portals being implemented by many cancer centers.

REFERENCES

Abernethy, A. P., L. M. Etheredge, P. A. Ganz, P. Wallace, R. R. German, C. Neti, P. B. Bach, and S. B. Murphy. 2010. Rapid-learning system for cancer care. *Journal of Clinical Oncology* 28(27):4268-4274.

Dalton, W. S., D. M. Sullivan, T. J. Yeatman, and D. A. Fenstermacher. 2010. The 2010 Health Care Reform Act: A potential opportunity to advance cancer research by taking cancer personally. *Clinical Cancer Research* 16(24):5987-5996.

Danaei, G., M. Tavakkoli, and M. A. Hernán. 2012. Bias in observational studies of prevalent users: Lessons for comparative effectiveness research from a meta-analysis of statins. *American Journal of Epidemiology* 175(4):250-262.

Fenstermacher, D. A., R. M. Wenham, D. E. Rollison, and W. S. Dalton. 2011. Implementing personalized medicine in a cancer center. *Cancer Journal* 17(6):528-536.

IOM (Institute of Medicine). 2010. *A foundation for evidence-driven practice: A rapid learning system for cancer care: Workshop summary.* Washington, DC: The National Academies Press.

NCI (National Cancer Institute). 2011. An assessment of the impact of the NCI Cancer Biomedical Informatics Grid (caBIG®). http://deainfo.nci.nih.gov/advisory/bsa/bsa0311/caBIGfinalReport.pdf (accessed July 11, 2012).

3

Informatics and Personalized Medicine

> **POINTS HIGHLIGHTED IN THE KEYNOTE ADDRESS BY LEROY HOOD**
>
> - The digital information of the genome and the environmental information that modifies the digital genomic information connect to produce the phenotype through biological networks.
> - A systems view of disease postulates that disease is the result of perturbation of one or more biological networks, leading to altered expression of information.
> - User-, domain-, and data-driven analytic informatics tools will allow researchers to decipher the billions of data points collected for an individual and use them to define and understand individual wellness and disease.
> - Together, systems biology and advanced informatics tools applied to disease and wellness provide the foundation for a personalized approach to medicine, allowing health care to be more predictive, preventive, personalized, and participatory.

Presenting the keynote address of the workshop, Leroy Hood, president and co-founder of the Institute for Systems Biology, shared his perspective on how the tremendous volumes of data currently becoming available can be utilized to advance medicine. An essential problem in biology in the 21st century is complexity, Hood said. He described his vision for the convergence of systems biology and the "digital revolution" to transform medicine into an enterprise that he has termed "proactive P4 medicine," in which P4 refers to predictive, preventive, personalized, and participatory.

Hood said that the digital revolution has provided three key elements that will play a central role in medicine going forward: (1) big datasets, (2) social and business networks that evolve from the knowledge gained from big datasets, and (3) digital personalized devices that will lead to the generation of a "quantized self."

Hood predicted that in 10 years, each individual will be surrounded by a virtual data cloud of billions of data points from many different types of networks (e.g., genome, proteome, transcriptome, epigenome, phenome, single cells, transactional, telehealth, social media). Big datasets have a lot of noise, and we must be able to analyze the individual types of data and put them into higher meta-level structures that will increase the signal and reduce the noise. Then we will be able to integrate these data to make predictive and actionable models to guide and inform health and medicine, he said.

AN INTEGRATIVE SYSTEMS APPROACH TO BIOLOGY, MEDICINE, AND COMPLEXITY

Biological complexity comes from the random and chaotic process of Darwinian evolution. Evolution arises from random mutations, is driven by environmental challenges, and selects solutions building on past successes, Hood said. To understand how a complex system achieves its end goal, one has to define all of the elements present, their interconnectivity, and their dynamics. This is the essence of systems biology.

Hood described his personal involvement in four paradigm changes that led him to the conceptualization of P4 medicine. First, bringing engineering to biology catalyzed high-throughput biology (e.g., instruments for automated sequencing and synthesizing genes and proteins). High-throughput biology, he noted, was the beginning of large datasets in biomedical research. Second, automated sequencing led to the human genome project, which democratized genes (i.e., made them available to all biologists) and created a complete gene "parts list" that was essential for systems biology. Making automated sequencing a reality required a chemist, an engineer, a computer scientist, and a biologist, and Hood realized that the futures of biology and technology were intertwined. For the third paradigm change, Hood founded the first cross-disciplinary university biology department to couple technology and analytic tool development to leading-edge biology research. Then, in 2000, he launched the first institute for the study of systems biology.

Simply stated, *systems biology* is a holistic and integrative approach to studying biological complexity, where frontier biology drives new technologies, which in turn catalyze novel domain-driven and data-driven computational tools; *systems medicine* is the application of the strategies, technologies, and computational tools of systems biology to disease and wellness; and *P4 medicine* is the clinical application of systems medicine to patients.

An integrated systems approach to disease is essential for dealing with complexity, Hood said, and he elaborated on the five pillars of that philosophy:

1. Viewing biology and medicine as *informational sciences* is one key to deciphering complexity.
2. *Systems biology infrastructure* involves a cross-disciplinary culture, democratization of data-generation and data-analysis tools, and the power of model organisms to decipher complexity.
3. *Holistic systems experimental approaches* enable deep insights into disease mechanisms and new approaches to diagnosis and therapy.
4. *Emerging technologies* enable large-scale data acquisition and permit exploration of new dimensions of patient data space.
5. *Transforming analytic tools* allow researchers to decipher the billions of data points for the individual, detailing wellness and disease.

Biology and Medicine as Informational Sciences

Human phenotypes are specified by two types of biological information: the digital information of the genome and the environmental information that modifies this digital information. These interact to generate the phenotype through biological networks that capture, transmit, process, and pass the information on to simple and complex molecular machines that execute the biological functions of life. Both the digital information and the environmental information are needed to understand how a system works. Hood pointed out that all levels of the biological information hierarchy—from DNA to RNA, proteins, interactions and networks, cells, organs, individuals, populations, and ecologies—are modified by environmental signals. If one wanted to understand the system at the level of the cell, for example, all of the preceding levels of information in the hierarchy would have to be captured and integrated in a way that can elucidate the contributions of the environmental signals in each of those steps.

Each technology will require a domain-driven software pipeline for acquisition, validation, storage, mining, integration, visualization, and modeling of data. Validation[1] is key, Hood stressed, and there currently are very few examples of good validation. In addition, different laboratories may not generate data that are interoperable, even if they use the same systems.

Systems Biology Infrastructure

Leading-edge biology research drives the development of technology and computation, facilitating the exploration of data in new dimensions, as well as a cycle of biological information (Figure 3-1). What is required for this cycle to be successful, Hood said, is a cross-disciplinary research environment, including biology, chemistry, computer science, engineering, mathematics, physics, and perhaps other disciplines, working together and communicating effectively in teams. A systems biology approach also facilitates democratization of the tools for data generation and analysis, so that any individual scientist can use them, regardless of the size of the project. This does not mean that every scientist has to learn how to do everything, Hood said, but there should be an environment that creates opportunities.

Holistic Systems Experimental Approaches

The systems approach to biology is holistic, seeking to understand how the individual components assemble and collectively create a functional whole. Hood used the analogy of a radio as a collection of individual transistors assembled onto circuit boards that together convert radio waves into sound waves. Human beings are essentially a collection of biological circuits and networks that process information into health or disease outcomes.

In an experimental systems biology approach, one creates a model from

---

[1] Validation refers to processes to ensure that the data are accurate and reproducible. Validation may also entail assessing an assay's measurement performance characteristics to determine the range of conditions under which the assay will give reproducible and accurate data (analytical validation), as well as assessing a test's ability to accurately and reliably predict the clinically defined disorder or phenotype of interest (clinical/biological validation).

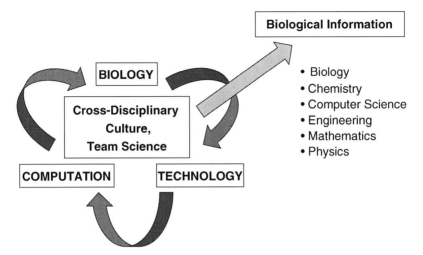

FIGURE 3-1 Systems biology infrastructure.
SOURCE: Hood presentation (February 27, 2012); Hood and Flores, 2012. Reprinted with permission from *New Biotechnology*.

extant data, formulates a hypothesis, and iteratively tests the model through experimental perturbations of the system. This can be both hypothesis driven and hypothesis generating and can produce large datasets. Experimental systems biology involves global analysis of all components (e.g., DNA, RNA, protein), evaluation of the dynamics of systems (both temporal and spatial), and integration of the different datasets from the system. Hood noted that large datasets are subject to two types of noise: technical noise resulting from how the data are acquired, managed, and analyzed and biological noise that arises as a natural consequence. Subtractive analysis can be used to help minimize biological noise. Ultimately, the goal is to convert data into knowledge.

A Systems View of Disease

A systems view of disease postulates that disease arises when one or more biological networks become perturbed, thereby altering the information they express. Systems medicine, Hood said, is really a network of networks. There are genetic networks at the level of the DNA, molecular networks at the level of proteins and other small molecules, cellular networks, organ networks, and social networks (Figure 3-2). We need to be able, from the various -omics data, to generate networks at each of these

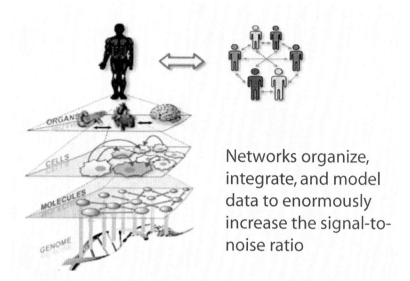

FIGURE 3-2 Systems medicine: A network of networks.
SOURCE: Hood presentation (February 27, 2012); Hood and Flores, 2012. Reprinted with permission from *New Biotechnology*.

levels and to integrate those networks to begin to understand the system. From a research perspective, networks are powerful ways of organizing, integrating, and modeling data, significantly increasing the signal-to-noise ratio. A systems approach to disease also allows the researcher to follow the disease from inception to end.

As an example, Hood described a systems approach to studying neurodegeneration in a mouse model. Briefly, inbred mice were injected with infectious prion particles and followed for changes in the transcriptome of their brains relative to the brains of normal littermates. Surprisingly, Hood and colleagues observed that 7,400 genes, or one-third of the mouse genome, were differentially expressed. The researchers then constructed eight combinations of inbred mouse strains and prion strains, carefully designed to exhibit different biologies that could be subtracted away. For example, one construct was a double knockout for the prion gene. When infectious prion particles were injected, the mice did not show signs of disease, but their brains underwent changes. Those changes that were not related to disease could be subtracted away. Subtractive transcriptome analysis based on this and the seven other mouse-prion strain combinations resulted in 300 differentially expressed genes. Subsequent serial histopathology identified four major disease-perturbed networks that played a major role in this prion disease process, and two-thirds of the genes mapped into these four networks. The remaining 100 genes defined six new networks that were previously unknown participants in prion disease. This is the power of global analyses, Hood said. There was also a sequential disease perturbation of all 10 of these networks, and the combined dynamics of these 10 networks can explain nearly all of the pathophysiology of prion disease (Hwang et al., 2009).

This study provided many new insights into potential biomarkers and diagnostics, Hood said. For example, he and his colleagues were able to demonstrate presymptomatic diagnosis of prion disease. They also established a fingerprint of the normal levels of 100 brain-specific proteins in human blood. The levels of proteins whose cognate networks become perturbed in disease will likely be altered in the blood, resulting in a unique fingerprint for each disease. Hood predicted that organ-specific blood proteins also will have utility for early disease detection, disease stratification, disease progression, following the progress of therapy, and assessing recurrences. Systems-driven blood-based diagnostics will be the key to P4 medicine, he said.

Emerging Technologies

Emerging technologies allow for large-scale data acquisition and analysis. Hood described four technology-driven projects with potential commercial applications on which the Institute for Systems Biology is currently working:

1. **Complete genome sequencing of families**—integrating genomics and genetics to find disease genes
2. **The Human Proteome Project**—selected reaction monitoring (SRM) mass spectrometry assays for all human proteins
3. **Clinical assays for patients**—allowing new dimensions of data space to be explored
4. **The Second Human Genome Project**—mining all complete human genomes and associated phenotypic or clinical data for the predictive medicine of the future

Family Genome Sequencing

The family genome sequencing project began with a family of two unaffected parents and two children each with genetic disease (Roach et al., 2010). By sequencing the genomes of a family of four and applying the principles of Mendelian genetics, one can identify 70 percent of the sequencing errors in the family, identify rare variants, determine the chromosomal haplotypes, determine the intergenerational mutation rate, and identify candidate genes for simple Mendelian diseases.

Hood predicted that within a decade, the human genome will be a part of every patient's medical record, and in 5 years, sequencing a human genome could cost as little as $100. He also predicted that any societal and scientific objections to routine genome sequencing will fade as actionable gene variants are identified. Every year, for example, patients could be checked for newly discovered actionable gene variants and provided with information that might be relevant to optimizing their health.

Hood added that the Institute for Systems Biology has developed a variety of software packages to manage the data from the family genomics project.

The Human Proteome Project

The Institute for Systems Biology pioneered four major advances that led to the consideration of a human proteome project, Hood explained. The first advance, the Trans Proteomic Pipeline, is a suite of software programs that validate mass spectrometry data. The software was developed using a bottom-up approach, driven by domain expertise and data. After validation, data are entered into the second new tool, the Peptide Atlas. The third new approach is targeted proteomics, which is the ability to use triple-quadrupole mass spectrometry to analyze 100 to 200 proteins in one hour. Finally, Hood and colleagues created targeted proteomic assays for most of the known 20,333 human proteins, and the results are being cataloged in the SRMAtlas database.

Moving forward, Hood suggested that the key clinical technology is not likely to be mass spectrometry but microfluidic protein chips. The Institute for Systems Biology, in collaboration with Caltech, currently has a prototype chip containing 50 ELISAs (enzyme-linked immunosorbent assays) that can be completed in about 5 minutes using 300 nanoliters of plasma. In the future, Hood would like to be able to assay 2,500 organ-specific blood proteins (50 from each of 50 organs) from millions of patients and follow them longitudinally to monitor wellness (as opposed to disease assessment) of each of those major organs.

Clinical Assays

Another focus of the Institute for Systems Biology is the development of individual patient information–based clinical assays. There are genomic and proteomic assays in development as well as single-cell analysis and induced pluripotent stem cells (iPS cells) for biology research and diagnostics development.

Single-cell analysis will impact the way we think about cancer, Hood said. For example, he observed quantitative transcriptome clustering of single cells from the human glioblastoma cell line U87. This is in contrast to a whole-tumor sequencing approach, where the signals of the individual cells are averaged and noise is enhanced. The reasons for this cellular heterogeneity are as yet unknown.

One ongoing project that Hood described involves differentiating iPS cells from healthy and diseased individuals into neurons, exposing them to environmental signals, and then using global and single-cell -omics analysis to try to understand the relative contributions of the digital genome and the environmental signals. Another example of the use of iPS cells is the stratification of complex genetic diseases such as Alzheimer's disease. The project involves creating iPS cells for each individual in the family of an affected individual; differentiating the cells into neurons; conducting single-cell analyses to identify and sort quantized cell states; exposing the sorted neuron populations to environmental probes such as drugs, ligands, or small interfering RNA (siRNA); and analyzing the transcriptome, select proteomes, microRNAome, etc. The intent is to stratify different subtypes of disease-perturbed networks and their response to environmental signals. The substratified populations of Alzheimer's patient cells could be provided to pharmaceutical companies to test the more than 100 drugs under investigation for Alzheimer's.

Domain-Driven, Transforming Analytic Tools

The last pillar of the integrative systems approach to disease that Hood described is the development of bottom-up, domain-driven analytic tools that will allow researchers to decipher the billions of data points collected for an individual and use them to define and understand individual wellness and disease. Hood mentioned The Cancer Genome Atlas (TCGA) as one example of genomic data integration and analysis. There are also efforts toward vertical integration, that is, integration of networks.

Hood advocated an open source platform for the development of software, suggesting that the advantages outweigh the challenges. In addition, he said software development should be driven by users, domain expertise, and data. Because of the complexity of biology, development needs to be bottom-up.

Hood highlighted several challenges to software development, including integrating biological expertise with statistical and computational expertise. Other challenges are integrating individual software packages or modules into coherent platforms for comprehensive modeling and determining the level of granularity of biological information that is needed.

APPLICATIONS OF SYSTEMS MEDICINE: THE P4 APPROACH

Together, systems biology and advanced informatics tools applied to disease and wellness provide the foundation for a personalized approach to medicine, allowing health care to be more predictive, preventive, personalized, and participatory. Hood outlined his perspectives and predictions about how a P4 approach to medicine could look in the future (Box 3-1).

Information Technology for Health Care

Information technology infrastructure is key to the advancement of P4 medicine, Hood said. There will be a need for sufficient infrastructure development and maintenance cycles; storage solutions for the vast amount of genomics, proteomics, and other data; and analytic tools that can access stored data from desktop platforms. Hood reiterated that systems should be open source, extensible, and interoperable, and the development of solutions should be domain expertise driven and data driven (i.e., bottom-up).

Among the technology and informatics challenges Hood listed were the lack of standards for electronic medical information; how to handle conventional medical records and histories as well as molecular, cellular, and phenotypic data; how to identify the actionable gene variants in individual genome sequences; and how to handle the comparative and subtractive analyses of billions of genomes and associated phenotypic data. Such challenges have also been noted by the President's Council of Advisors on

BOX 3-1
P4 Medicine: Perspectives from Leroy Hood on What the Future Could Hold

Predictive

- In 10 years, most individuals will have had their genome sequenced.
- Genomic information will be used to design probabilistic health history, a lifelong strategy that will optimize individual wellness and manage the potential for disease.
- Individuals will have regular, multiparameter blood measurements done, assaying perhaps up to 2,500 organ-specific blood proteins at once, to predict any transition from health into disease and facilitate a timely response.

Preventive

- Taking a systems medicine approach, therapeutic and preventive drugs and vaccines will be developed to modify disease-perturbed networks so that they operate in a more normal fashion.
- Maintaining wellness (rather than treatment of disease) will increasingly be the focus of medicine.

Personalized

- Individuals are genetically unique, differing by 6 million nucleotides from one another.
- Each patient will serve as his or her own control for analysis of the vast, longitudinal datasets that will be generated.

Participatory

- The patient will become the center of the P4 health care network, and patient-driven social networks for disease and wellness will be a driving force for change.
- Society should be able to access patient data after de-identification and make them available to biologists for pioneering the predictive medicine approaches of the future.
- Patients, physicians, and other members of the health care community will have to be educated about P4 medicine so they can participate fully.

SOURCE: Hood presentation (February 27, 2012).

Science and Technology (PCAST) in its recent report on the use of health information technology to improve health care (PCAST, 2010).

The digital revolution will generate enormous amounts of useful personal data including, for example, imaging data, longitudinal data, and social network data, existing together in a dynamic "network of networks," Hood concluded. There will have to be ways to integrate all of these data into predictive models and actionable opportunities, he said.

REFERENCES

Hood, L., and M. Flores. 2012. A personal view on systems medicine and the emergence of proactive P4 medicine: Predictive, preventive, personalized and participatory. *New Biotechnology* March 18. [Epub ahead of print].

Hwang, D., I. Y. Lee, H. Yoo, N. Gehlenborg, J. H. Cho, B. Petritis, D. Baxter, R. Pitstick, R. Young, D. Spicer, N. D. Price, J. G. Hohmann, S. J. Dearmond, G. A. Carlson, and L. E. Hood. 2009. A systems approach to prion disease. *Molecular Systems Biology* 5:252.

PCAST (President's Council of Advisors on Science and Technology). 2010. *Report to the President: Realizing the full potential of health information technology to improve healthcare for all Americans: The path forward.* http://www.whitehouse.gov/sites/default/files/microsites/ostp/pcast-health-it-report.pdf (accessed July 10, 2012).

Roach, J. C., G. Glusman, A. F. Smit, C. D. Huff, R. Hubley, P. T. Shannon, L. Rowen, K. P. Pant, N. Goodman, M. Bamshad, J. Shendure, R. Drmanac, L. B. Jorde, L. Hood, and D. J. Galas. 2010. Analysis of genetic inheritance in a family quartet by whole-genome sequencing. *Science* 328(5978):636-639.

4

Informatics-Supported Cancer Research Endeavors

> **DISCUSSION POINTS HIGHLIGHTED BY INDIVIDUAL PRESENTERS**
>
> - Cloud-based informatics platforms aim to simplify interaction and information sharing between scientists and oncologists so that targeted treatments can begin faster; can manage billions of data points generated per patient; and can reduce time for data mapping and analysis from months to days to create a real-time, growing body of knowledge.
> - The National Comprehensive Cancer Network (NCCN) outcomes database is one example of a collaborative data collection system that is relevant to both clinical practice and robust clinical outcomes research.
> - Web-based EHR systems can facilitate real-time alerts, decision support capability, and multiple user applications.
> - Patient-centered outcomes empower providers to make tailored recommendations to the individual patient based on data from other patients most like them.
> - Secondary use of data that were collected for a different primary purpose generally involves some sort of adaptation or compromise. The challenge is to identify how this secondary use can best complement and extend the primary use of the data, for example, for generation of new hypotheses.
>
> *continued*

> - Trust is the core underlying issue for concerns regarding consent, data privacy and security, accountability, and data ownership. Consumers and patients want their data to be protected, and they want medicine and health care to be advanced.

In this session, four cancer use cases were presented as examples of successful informatics-supported approaches to managing large, complex datasets. Panelists discussed data collection, storage, and retrieval; data analysis and reporting; and data sharing.

CASE EXAMPLE: DELL-TGen CLOUD COMPUTING COLLABORATION IN PERSONALIZED MEDICINE FOR PEDIATRIC NEUROBLASTOMA

Spyro Mousses, vice president in the Office of Innovation and director of the Center for BioIntelligence at the Translational Genomics Research Institute (TGen), described a clinical trial using molecularly guided individualized therapy in pediatric cancer as a case example of successful alignment of biomedical science and informatics. To begin, Mousses described what he called "the evolution from evidence-based medicine to information-enabled medicine to intelligence-based medicine" and TGen's "$N = 1$" approach to drug development (Figure 4-1).

An $N = 1$ Approach to Clinical Research

When seeking to develop a drug for a deadly disease such as cancer, investigators generally start with a broad target population from which they select a representative study cohort for a clinical trial comparing one therapeutic option against another. Evidence-based decisions on treatment are informed by statistical outcomes of the trial. For example, if the data indicate a 30 percent response rate to therapeutic option 1 and a 20 percent response rate to option 2, then therapeutic option 1 would be the drug of choice to be developed for all patients in the original target population (Figure 4-1A). Such a statistical approach is not ideal when dealing with a disease or condition that is clinically heterogeneous and molecularly complex, Mousses said.

Moving beyond basic evidence-based medicine, information-enabled

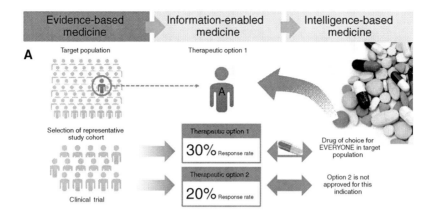
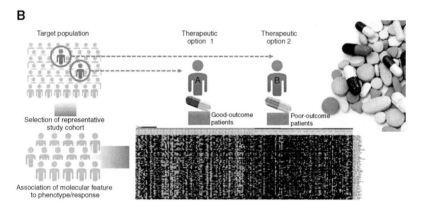
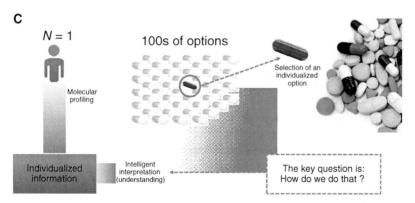

FIGURE 4-1 The evolution from evidence-based medicine (A) to information-enabled medicine (B) to intelligence-based medicine (C).
SOURCE: Mousses presentation (February 27, 2012).

medicine takes into account more detailed characteristics of the disease, such as expression of tumor markers or measurement of biomarkers. This approach also starts with a target population and the selection of a representative cohort for a clinical trial, but the cohort is then further stratified based on the association of a molecular feature with a phenotype or response. This stratification can allow one to determine that patient A would benefit more from therapeutic option 1, while patient B would be better treated with therapeutic option 2 (Figure 4-1B). Still, there are affected individuals who do not respond to either drug A or drug B.

To help address these concerns, TGen has been experimenting with an N of 1 approach where the focus is not on finding a representative population in which to test an investigative compound, but rather on finding a drug that meets the needs of a single individual based on his or her molecular profile (Figure 4-1C). This approach requires intelligent interpretation of individualized information and a mechanistic understanding of the disease to allow for predictions about which therapy is most appropriate. About a decade ago, TGen started to take the fundamental steps in the direction of molecular-based cancer treatments and has been using technologies ranging from simple gene expression and chemical assays to whole-genome sequencing to identify targets, Mousses said.

Molecularly Guided Individualized Cancer Therapy

As an example of the N of 1 approach to drug development, Mousses described an ongoing pediatric neuroblastoma clinical trial. To make the most of its molecular technologies, TGen needed innovative IT infrastructure. Through a collaboration with Dell, it created a cloud-based computing system that would both support the workflow of the trial and aid in repurposing the data. It is both a cloud to support personalized medicine, Mousses explained, and a repository to support translational research. As a result, the trial will be expanding to other pediatric and young adult cancers.

The process starts with clinical trial design, working within the framework of the regulatory agencies and in accordance with the IRBs. Following consent and enrollment of the patients, biopsies are collected and molecular profiling is done using next-generation sequencing technologies. Mousses noted that the collaboration with Dell has allowed faster and deeper profiling for each child and faster and improved data and clinical communication. A personalized treatment plan is then devised based on the profiling. This model for personalized medicine clinical trials, using molecularly guided treatment and the Dell IT infrastructure and TGen cloud, is also being used for a new melanoma trial.

These types of trials are necessary experiments, Mousses said, to help define the IT requirements for intelligence-based personalized medicine using cloud-based informatics. The molecular profiling presents the first IT challenge, requiring high-performance computing and storage for 200 billion data points generated per patient. Another IT challenge is to match the patient profile to known information about therapeutic concepts, pathway concepts, and cellular processes, for example. This requires very large knowledge databases (e.g., pharmacogenomic databases) and presents numerous challenges. How should these complex, heterogeneous data be presented and processed? How can they be shared and exchanged across sites? There are also issues of security and privacy in the cloud. One of the models TGen is exploring is a hybrid cloud, where each clinical center would be able to warehouse its own data, keeping the patient data secure within the confines of the health care enterprise.

Opportunities in the Cloud

The TGen model for personalized medicine clinical trials facilitates intelligent use of the data to help each individual patient, Mousses said, but it does not yet allow for repurposing the data for secondary studies. TGen's future vision is to provide a system that effectively links the pediatric oncology community, including software, hardware, and protocols that support data exchanges so that they are secure. Infrastructure for communication and collaboration is critical, Mousses said, and the system would include scientific, clinical, and community web portals. The goal is for the wider oncology community to have access to the network and be able to manage, analyze, and link patient data to pharmacological knowledge to identify potential treatment options. Information about the prediction and the outcome should feed into the model to create a real-time growing body of knowledge, not just about what is working, but about what is not working as well.

August Calhoun, vice president at Dell Healthcare and Life Sciences Services, added that the cloud increases computation and collaboration capacity by 1,200 percent and reduces the time needed for data mapping and analysis from months to days. The cloud is a shared resource that will be accessed over the Internet to do the complex analyses required to make better-informed decisions about care and to share information in a consented and secure manner, he said.

CASE EXAMPLE: NATIONAL COMPREHENSIVE CANCER NETWORK OUTCOMES DATABASE

NCCN is an affiliation of 21 leading cancer centers throughout the United States. The overarching mission of the network, explained Kimary Kulig, vice president of clinical and translational outcomes research at NCCN, is to improve the quality, effectiveness, and efficiency of oncology practice so that patients can live better lives. NCCN seeks to enhance care through information resources, outcomes research, and clinical trials, and to develop information resources that are valuable to patients and other stakeholders within the health care delivery system.

NCCN Guidelines

To aid in fulfilling its mission, NCCN issues comprehensive oncology clinical practice guidelines that include clinical algorithms and supporting documentation for various tumor types. There are currently 56 individual guidelines covering 97 percent of all malignant diseases. Guidelines are developed and continually updated in collaboration with the 21 NCCN member institutions and efforts that involve more than 18,000 volunteer-hours per year from 900 clinicians who participate on guideline panels. Guidelines are categorized according to both level of evidence and degree of consensus among panel members.

NCCN Oncology Outcomes Database

To understand the extent to which NCCN member institutions adhered to the guidelines they helped to develop, NCCN launched an outcomes database. In addition to the primary goals of monitoring and benchmarking concordance with the guidelines, the database was also intended to be used to describe patterns and outcomes of care under the guidelines and to create a feedback loop to the physicians, institutions, and guideline panel members. Kulig noted that the outcomes database has also become a major data repository for research, aided by the fact that it is based on a common data dictionary and thus serves as a platform for multi-institutional health services research.

The first database, launched in 1997, was focused on breast cancer and currently includes data on close to 54,000 patients who are followed actively throughout their entire course of treatment until death. There are 17 institutions actively participating in this database. With the architecture in place, databases for other tumor types were subsequently launched, including non-Hodgkin's lymphoma, colorectal cancer, non-small-cell lung cancer, and ovarian cancer.

Structure and Operations

The NCCN outcomes database is governed by the Scientific Office, a virtual office that includes investigators who are chairs of each of the tumor-specific databases. The data coordinating center is housed at the City of Hope Cancer Center in Los Angeles, California, and clinical research associates at each participating center abstract and de-identify the data for submission to a centralized, web-based database. Kulig noted that this is done under an IRB-approved protocol in every site and that most of the IRBs now have a waiver of consent unless the patient's data are linked to specimen collection protocols. The patients included in the database have received all or most of their care at an NCCN institution, and each patient is followed longitudinally throughout the course of care (Kulig added that outside medical records are unfortunately not accessed for abstraction in this database). The NCCN main office in Fort Washington, Pennsylvania, employs project managers, quality assurance managers, statisticians, and analysts who work with the aggregate data from all of the databases and all of the sites.

There are some unique characteristics of the NCCN outcomes database, Kulig said, that differentiate it from other large datasets (e.g., the Surveillance, Epidemiology, and End Results Program [SEER]) or other institutional databases. The NCCN database has more than 300 different data elements that track the continuum of care for each patient. There is complete data on patient demographics, medical histories, family histories, and comorbidities. Detailed information about sites of metastases and biomarkers is also collected. All clinical events and interventions are collected, including diagnostics, hospital admissions, very detailed sequencing of therapies, and reasons for discontinuation of chemotherapy. Progression-free and overall survival data are also captured.

Kulig contrasted this to tumor registry data, which generally contain no information on comorbidity or diagnostic procedures and only limited data on treatment and outcomes (limited to recurrence and survival data). She also drew a contrast to claims or billing data, which are not research-quality data to begin with; which have no information on staging, pathology, or histology; and from which treatment data can be very difficult to interpret. There is generally no biomarker information, and the outcome end points that can be derived from billing or claims data are usually in the form of resource utilization to which costs can be affixed.

NCCN has rigorous data quality assurance processes in place, starting with extensive data manager training. The system also includes online edit checking during web-based entry, programmed logic checks (e.g., flagging an entry if a prostate cancer patient is entered as female), quarterly quality assurance reports, and on-site audits.

Five NCCN sites are currently using electronic data transfer for the breast cancer database, Kulig said. This is particularly important at high-volume sites to maximize efficiencies (e.g., eliminates the need to enter the same data multiple times into various databases, such as the tumor registry, the NCCN database, or any internal databases). Electronic data transfer does need dedicated resources, including programming support to conform to the NCCN database requirements and changes. Lack of dedicated resources can lead to failed audits or poor-quality data, Kulig said. The fact that some sites are using electronic data transfer while others are not does add complexity to the system, and every proposed change by NCCN must be carefully considered for how it will affect electronic data transfer sites versus manual data entry sites.

Current Use

The primary use of the NCCN outcomes database is the annual analysis of institutional concordance to the NCCN guidelines. This is done systematically for each tumor database, comparing the care that was actually received in practice to the guideline that was in effect at the time the care was delivered. (Kulig noted that any treatment received as part of a clinical trial is considered concordant.) Each institution's care is then benchmarked against the NCCN aggregate, and individual reports are provided to each institution for quality-improvement purposes. Individual patient summary reports can be generated from the database and are useful for viewing concordance status, treatment information, or visit history, for example.

The database is also very conducive to comparative effectiveness research, Kulig said, because it contains detailed information about the patient's clinical characteristics, comorbidities, and treatment. Institution-specific data are available to NCCN sites, and aggregate data are available upon request. The data are also available to non-NCCN entities for specific research queries, and Kulig noted that NCCN has provided data to pharmaceutical, biotechnology, information technology, and medical device companies.

Value of Collaborative Databases for Diverse Stakeholders

When we think of the continuum of data and how it is generated, Kulig said, controlled clinical trial data provide the strongest evidence for safety, efficacy, and even patient-reported outcomes. Such high-quality data can also provide information about the predictive and prognostic value of diagnostic testing and biomarkers.

Beyond the clinical trial, Kulig suggested, a lot of observational data generated every day in clinical practice is often underutilized or even ignored, including real-world safety and effectiveness data; patient-reported preferences and outcomes; adherence to, duration of, and reasons for discontinuation of therapy; biomarkers and diagnostic testing; and resource use and costs of care. A variety of stakeholders make use of real-world data for a variety of purposes (Box 4-1).

Personalized medicine has a particular need for real-world, real-time data. Kulig noted that lags in existing datasets, the NCCN dataset included, do not necessarily accommodate real-time analysis or cutting-edge biomarker-linked outcomes research. In addition, there are large biospecimen repositories in numerous institutions that are not necessarily annotated or linked to clinical data.

In conclusion, Kulig said, the NCCN outcomes database is one example of a collaborative data collection system that is relevant to both clinical practice and robust clinical outcomes research. Observational, real-world data hold value for key stakeholders. The promise of personalized medicine in particular underscores the need for these types of data aggregation and exchange systems.

CASE EXAMPLE: IT INNOVATIONS FOR COMMUNITY CANCER PRACTICES

Cancer costs are rising more rapidly than inflation and other health care costs, and community cancer centers are facing more challenges than ever, said Asif Ahmad, senior vice president for information and technology

> **BOX 4-1**
> **What Real-World Data Are Used by Whom?**
>
> *Clinicians*
> - Treatment effectiveness
> - Adverse events and safety
>
> *Food and Drug Administration*
> - Epidemiology
> - Adverse events and safety
>
> *Payers*
> - Adverse events and safety
> - Comparative effectiveness
> - Resource use and costs
>
> *Patients and Caregivers*
> - Treatment effectiveness; real-world survival
> - Adverse events and safety, symptoms and side effects, quality of life
> - Costs of care
>
> *Manufacturers*
> - Epidemiology, current practice patterns, unmet medical need
> - Treatment effectiveness versus comparators; real-world survival
> - Side effects and adverse events, hospitalizations, resource use and costs
>
> SOURCE: Kulig presentation (February 27, 2012).

services at McKesson Specialty Health. McKesson Specialty Health partners with community cancer care practices to help them manage increased competition from hospitals and clinics, declines in reimbursement, health care reform uncertainty, and rising health care costs. McKesson Specialty Health is the second-largest business unit of McKesson, which is one of the largest distributors of specialty pharmaceuticals and biologics. The company has long-term partnerships with about 3,000 oncologists, about 1,000 of whom are in the U.S. Oncology Network, and 2,200 multispecialty practices.

Ahmad said that the foundation of McKesson Specialty Health is IT, upon which is built the robust customer-facing technology from which analytic applications stem. The customers could be patients, pharmaceutical manufacturers, payers, or others. The focus is on developing an efficient, integrated technology suite built upon the core architecture.

System Design and Datasets

The cornerstone of the McKesson system is the iKnowMed Electronic Health Record, one of the first totally hosted, web-based EHR systems, Ahmad said. iKnowMed includes charge capture functionality, safety alerts to help decrease errors, a cancer diagnosis and regimen library to aid point-of-care decision making, and clinical trial support to help increase clinical trial accruals. It integrates with other tools such as oral e-prescribing and drug inventory management. One benefit for practices is the ability to drive the workflow of the clinic from a single place. Another unique feature of the system is the support for real-time decision making. Ahmad added that all of the data feed into a common data management system that currently warehouses data for about 1.2 million patients, with 17,000 newly diagnosed cancer patients added to the McKesson database every month.

Ahmad reiterated that the customer-facing technology is all built upon the same structural data framework. For example, data in the common core framework could be used for real-time clinical alerts that could inform the clinician about a newly diagnosed patient for the purposes of clinical trial recruitment or alert the nurse to a scheduled appointment for a patient coming for the first dose of treatment. The same technology drives alerts for pharmaceutical manufacturers that may include aggregate, de-identified data regarding use of their products. The CARE, or Comprehensive Accrual REsource, tool for clinical research is also built on the same technology and facilitates identification of patients for personalized medicine trials. The same data framework is used to pull up the weekly and monthly financial reports for the practices. Rather than duplicating efforts, everything comes from one source. That data store is fed by the EHR, practice management tools, and patient-reported data from the patient portal. Ahmad noted that the technology architecture is able to use data from whatever practice management tools the practice has chosen to use.

Supporting Clinical Outcomes and Research

Current trends in health care reform, consumerism, pay for performance, and care delivery models are changing the landscape of medical practice. The old model of "patient plus prescription results in payment" is being replaced with one where demonstrated outcomes impact payment. The McKesson system allows researchers to harness clinical data to show cost-effectiveness of care alongside evidence for best possible outcomes. Another feature is the ability to provide a market intelligence report to manufacturers, which can show, for example, the penetration of a particular drug in the market compared to a competitor. The same data are integrated with the clinical trial management system, Ahmad said; this has facilitated the enrollment of more than 50,000 patients in various clinical trials over the past 8 years.

Data Governance

Because no defined standards are fully implemented with regard to EHRs, the data remain somewhat "dirty," Ahmad said. To help address this, McKesson established a multidisciplinary data governance committee tasked with increasing stakeholder awareness of the importance of data quality and working collaboratively with all stakeholders to ensure the accuracy, completeness, and consistency of the clinical, administrative, and financial data that are entered into the database. The committee will consider data governance from a very comprehensive point of view, including, for example, common definitions, structure and standardization, data validation, data access and compliance with regulations, communication, prioritization, and benchmarks.

CASE EXAMPLE: SECONDARY USES OF DATA FOR COMPARATIVE EFFECTIVENESS RESEARCH

Paul Wallace, senior vice president and director of the Center for Comparative Effectiveness Research at The Lewin Group, a health care and health policy consultancy in Washington, DC, began with a brief overview of the evolution of comparative effectiveness research.

Comparative effectiveness research (CER) was defined in the Medicare Modernization Act of 2003 as "the conduct and synthesis of research comparing the benefits and harms of different interventions and strategies to prevent, diagnose, treat and monitor health conditions in 'real world' settings." Subsequently, the Agency for Healthcare Research and Quality (AHRQ) created programs to foster CER, and in 2009, the American Recovery and Reinvestment Act (ARRA) provided $1.1 billion to fund CER. The Patient Protection and Affordable Care Act of 2010 included further provisions to foster CER, including the creation of the Patient-Centered Outcomes Research Institute (PCORI). Chartered as an independent, nonprofit research organization with a sustainable funding stream, PCORI's charge is to fund research that offers patients and caregivers the information they need to make important health care decisions.

Patient-centered outcomes research is a relatively new term, Wallace explained, and there has been some tension as to what it is and what it is not, as well as how it contrasts with personalized medicine. According to the PCORI working definition, patient-centered outcomes research

> helps people and their caregivers communicate and make informed health care decisions, allowing their voices to be heard in assessing the value of health care options. This research answers patient-centered questions such as: Given my personal characteristics, conditions, and preferences, what should I expect will happen to me? What are my options and what are the potential benefits and harms of those options? What can I do to improve the outcomes that are most important to me? How can clinicians and the care delivery systems they work in help me make the best decisions about my health and health care? (PCORI, 2012).

Wallace added that from a practice perspective, patient-centered outcomes research will empower the oncologist to have more robust conversations with an individual patient about what is known about similar patients, how his or her situation compares and relates to others, and how the patient and practitioner can move forward on the basis of that information.

The draft research agenda recently released by PCORI indicates that 20 percent of funding will be allocated to accelerating patient-centered outcomes research and to methodological research, particularly for conducting observational research, Wallace said. There has been an evolution in how evidence is perceived (Table 4-1). Expert opinion based on case reports and case series is still important and credible, but it is based on chart review and clinician experience (essentially an N of 1). Evidence-based medicine is more from the perspective of population efficacy (an N of many). Data from clinical trials and systematic reviews are expressed as a mean, and subgroups of people are thereby excluded. While population efficacy is translated into a variety of practices, from performance management to

TABLE 4-1 The Evolving Evidence Perspective

Study Type	Methods	Data Source/Organization	Perspective
Expert Opinion	• Case Reports • Case Series	• Charts • Experience	Effects on Patients (N of 1)
Evidence-Based Medicine	• RCTs • Systematic Reviews • (Observation)	• Trial Data & Databases • Meta-analysis • Reports & Series	Population Efficacy (N of Many)
Comparative Effectiveness Research	• RCTs • Systematic Reviews • Observation	• Trial Data & Databases • Meta-analysis • Large Population Databases • Reports & Series	Population Effectiveness (N of Many)
Patient-Centered Outcomes Research	• RCTs • Systematic Reviews • Systematic Observation	• Trial Data & Databases • Meta-analysis • Large Population Databases • Reports & Series • Patient-Generated Data	Patient Effectiveness (Many N of 1s)

NOTE: RCT = randomized clinical trial.
SOURCE: Wallace presentation (February 27, 2012).

guidelines, Wallace noted that there are pitfalls, not the least of which is that the data may not be particularly applicable to the individual patient in the room. Comparative effectiveness research uses large population databases to consider population effectiveness (also an N of many). The key difference between evidence-based medicine and CER, Wallace suggested, is that CER attempts to include those groups of people who were ineligible for and excluded from clinical trials, using observational data to complement and extend what was learned from the trial. Patient-centered outcomes research builds on all of the previously discussed dimensions, focusing on patient effectiveness (many N of 1s). In other words, what is the provider's recommendation to the individual patient, based on as many people like that patient as can be found?

Secondary Use of Data

When considering "secondary use" of data, Wallace said, it is important to remember that this means the intended primary use was most likely for a different purpose and the data were collected under different rules. As a result, secondary use of data generally involves some sort of adaptation or compromise. The challenge is to identify how this secondary use can best complement and extend the primary use of the data. Wallace outlined several approaches to secondary use.

Most secondary uses have been reactive and opportunistic, making use of any data that are already there. Wallace mentioned the Optum Natural History of Disease (NHD) Model as an example of how data can be used for secondary analysis. Using claims data, this application can answer questions such as, How many people within a population are taking a particular lipid drug and how do they differ from matched people with the same clinical situation who are not taking the same drug? While it would take about a year and a half to answer that question by going through charts, Wallace said, the NHD applications could answer within minutes, making use of big datasets that are optimally structured. Reactive secondary analysis can be useful for forming new hypotheses or for iterative testing to refine a hypothesis.

A different approach is to plan for secondary use. This may involve structured data capture, expanded common datasets outside clinical trials, or common intervention protocols. Planning for secondary analysis can help to answer questions that cannot be answered by classical experimental approaches. For example, What are the drivers from the patient side for choosing to undertake a third line of therapy? Can differences in costs and response rates for various lines of therapy be demonstrated? How do survival and costs for advanced cancer patients who opt not to have therapy compare to those who are treated?

Wallace cited a variety of ongoing efforts in secondary use of data that support CER and patient-centered outcomes research, including the FDA Sentinel system that uses data to track the safety of products on the market and the National Institute of Mental Health (NIMH) Registry of Individuals with Autism Spectrum Disorders to test hypotheses about etiology and health services use by patients and families.

Sustainability

The sustainability of these projects is an ongoing challenge, Wallace concluded. There is a necessary balance and overlap between funding and governance, and between data sources and data users. Surrounding this are issues regarding the use of distributed versus aggregated data, cost structure for participation, preservation of privacy and confidentiality, and proprietary and ownership issues.

CROSS-CUTTING ISSUES

Following the presentation of case examples, a reaction panel moderated by Adam Clark, patient advocacy consultant at MedTran Health Strategies, discussed further some of the cross-cutting issues for informatics-supported cancer research and care. Panelists included Gwen Darien, director of the Pathways Project and cancer survivor, Deven McGraw, director of the Health Privacy Project at the Center for Democracy and Technology, James Cimino, chief of the NIH Laboratory for Informatics Development, and Steven Piantadosi, director of the Samuel Oschin Comprehensive Cancer Institute at Cedars-Sinai Medical Center.

Engaging Patients

Gwen Darien offered the patient's perspective based on both her personal experience as a cancer survivor and input from her colleagues in the advocacy community. The advocacy community is not as engaged in health IT and informatics as it needs to be, she said. To create buy-in and engagement of the survivor advocacy community, that community should be engaged from the beginning, during the conceptualizing of the process and parameters of information exchange (rather than simply participating afterward). Are patients people that something is done to, she asked, or are they active partners in the formulation and creation of value? Data are an asset. What is the value of patients to health IT, and what do the patients get out of sharing their data in return? Who owns the information and what information do patients have access to?

Darien noted that a barrier to moving forward in informatics is the broad assumptions made about "the patient." Some patients are extremely engaged, some disengage once their treatment is over, others do not want to know anything.

Building Trust: Privacy, Consent, and Ownership

Deven McGraw said that the end goal of privacy is not privacy itself, but trust. The goal is to build a trusted, accountable ecosystem for using data in ways that help individuals, communities, and populations. Privacy rules are structured largely around tools such as patient consent and data minimization or de-identification. These tools are critically important, McGraw said, but they are not the end goal. They are tools to be used to build trust, along with other tools. It is also important to remember that consumers and patients want their data to be protected, and they want medicine and health care to be advanced. These competing interests need to be considered and balanced when developing privacy policies.

McGraw also suggested that too much time is spent focusing just on the issue of consent in lieu of addressing other important privacy protections. Consent is not the same as privacy. Consent ends up shifting the burden for protecting privacy to the patient. That said, when surveyed, people often say that they want to be asked before their data are used for research purposes. There are efforts now to obtain general consent for future research because it is not possible to define all of the potential research uses of the data being collected today, but this does not lead to a meaningful and informed consent for the patient, she said. Building trust in research requires research institutions to be mindful of the sensitivity of the data, to treat them with respect, and to make good decisions about how the data are to be used. McGraw suggested that one of the ways to rely less on consent and build trust is to improve transparency, both to the public at large and to cancer patients, about how patient data are used, the typical tools that institutions use to protect data, and oversight and accountability for those protections.

Consent as a policy issue is also important for researchers because their access to clinical data is based on informed consent. James Cimino pointed out that if the data are going to be reused in de-identified form, the original investigators are notified of reuse. This raises the issue of the ownership of the data and goes beyond the patient or the institution to the intellectual property of the investigators who are providing these data for sharing.

Workshop participant Alison Smith from C-Change asked what role additional penalties for inappropriate and irresponsible use of data played in the trust equation. McGraw expressed her concern that imposing penalties and creating the threat of legal liability can cause people to be unwilling to share data, because that is the path of least risk. Regulators need to do more than impose penalties, she said; they need to provide more guidance about how to comply with HIPAA Privacy Rule (IOM, 2009).

Data Granularity

James Cimino highlighted several technical issues of data granularity in databases. When repositories collect data from different sources, one of the concerns is determining when the data collected are synonymous and when are they not. The level of data granularity in clinical care is not necessarily the same as the level of granularity in research data (e.g., noting the patient had pain versus reporting the severity of pain on a scale of 1 to 10 and where exactly the pain was). Capturing the context of the data is also important (e.g., was a complete blood count done because the patient had a fever, or was it part of the protocol data collection schedule?). Another technical aspect is the inclusion of genomic data. What is important to index? How can the system cope with the changing methods of how these data are being collected?

Secondary Use

Steven Piantadosi added his perspective as a clinical trialist. Expanding on the comments by Wallace, he stressed that data that are intended and designed to address a particular therapeutic question are distinct from data that were produced for some other purpose. He urged caution when making inferences based on data that were not collected for that purpose. One example is when a safety signal emerges in a clinical trial designed to consider a therapeutic question. Even in a highly structured clinical protocol, it can be very difficult to determine whether or not the safety signal is real and actionable when the study was not designed specifically to study it. These are not new issues, and for historical perspective, Piantadosi referred participants to a 1984 article discussing the use of observational data from registries to make treatment comparisons (Green and Byar, 1984).

Kulig added that observational data are largely underutilized because of concerns from both a statistical and a clinical perspective. Wallace said that just because we do not have statistically significant data does not mean we do not make decisions. While the foundation of decision making is ideally experimental empirical data, there are many questions for which empirical data will not exist. Frameworks are needed that can help clinicians make progressively better care decisions for each individual patient, even in the absence of gold standard data. Piantadosi suggested that it is not a question of having the perfect data source, but rather a problem of bias. These databases are not unbiased sources of information on which to base definitive statements about therapeutic decisions. Mousses concurred that we should not be making definitive statements about something that the data were not generated to address in the first place. The data can be mined, aggregated, and used to identify trends and design studies to test new hypotheses, he said. There may be bias in the data, but there may be a signal nonetheless that could guide further study.

Engaging Private Practice and Extramural Researchers

Piantadosi noted that the majority of faculty at Cedars-Sinai are in private practice (i.e., not employed directly by the hospital) and it is difficult to incentivize them appropriately with regard to informatics needs. If, as was noted earlier, 80 percent of patients are treated outside of academic centers, we have to find ways to incentivize the private practice community to use the tools and provide the data that are needed, he said.

Clark asked what would be needed for the governance or implementation of an interconnected system that would engage community practices in data exchange. One solution, Piantadosi said, is to buy the practice. Independent practices tend to see things in terms of time spent and cost, and they do not respond well to edicts from the parent institution. Practitioners may also be less computer savvy, either because of their background or the nature of the practice.

Cimino said that NIH intramural investigators are being encouraged to collaborate extramurally, and the clinical center is opening its doors to extramural investigators to bring in their patients for studies and to make use of some of the unique resources that NIH has. With regard to governance, there is currently no coordinated trans-institute effort to share data within or outside NIH, other than what individual researchers choose to do. The IT working group of an advisory council to the NIH director is considering how to better coordinate intramural and extramural work, and a report is expected in 2012.

REFERENCES

Green, S. B., and D. P. Byar. 1984. Using observational data from registries to compare treatments: The fallacy of omnimetrics. *Statistics in Medicine* 3(4):361-373.

IOM (Institute of Medicine). 2009. *Beyond the HIPAA privacy rule: Enhancing privacy, improving health through research*. Washington, DC: The National Academies Press.

PCORI (Patient-Centered Outcomes Research Institute). 2012. *Patient-centered outcomes research*. http://www.pcori.org/patient-centered-outcomes-research/ (accessed April 26, 2012).

5

Potential Pathways and Models for Moving Forward

**DISCUSSION POINTS HIGHLIGHTED
BY INDIVIDUAL PRESENTERS**

- Volumes of molecular, clinical, and epidemiological data already exist in thousands of data repositories. Integrating data that are already in the public domain to generate new hypotheses for testing can help to identify new diagnostics, therapeutics, and disease mechanisms.
- An integrated knowledge ecosystem that supports moving data from discovery to actionable intelligence could drive better decision making and a learning health care enterprise.
- The overarching biomedical informatics challenges are systems issues; scale, standards, and sharing; software, storage, and security; sustainability; and social issues (changing mindsets and behaviors).
- Convenience and personal empowerment drive the disruptive innovation in service industries, and this will be the case for health care as well, with the patient or consumer as a primary disrupter.
- Numerous end-user applications can be developed on a core enterprise analytics platform, allowing researchers, clinicians, administrators, and others to analyze high-quality data. A common infrastructure can also support secondary uses of data.

To set the stage for discussion in the third panel session, John Mendelsohn, Forum chair, highlighted some of the key needs identified thus far in the speaker presentations. One main area of concern was the collection, structure, storage, and analysis of big datasets, including the need for interoperability and standardization of systems. In addition, observational research requires that the data be de-identified and pooled. Mendelsohn noted that the more technical issues of computer power, software, and interconnectivity did not seem to be major concerns.

Another main area of discussion was data scrutiny and use, which are affected by ethical and social issues more than scientific issues. Key issues raised by individual participants were patient privacy and trust. Many stakeholders need or want access to the data, including patients themselves, investigators, universities, pharmaceutical companies, the government, and others. There are questions of whether there is ownership of the data and, if so, by whom.

With these needs and concerns in mind, panelists discussed a variety of approaches for moving the field of cancer informatics forward.

PUBLIC DATA-DRIVEN SYSTEMS AND PERSONALIZED MEDICINE

Atul Butte, chief of the Division of Systems Medicine at Stanford University and Lucile Packard Children's Hospital, shared examples of how public data can drive science and enable personalized medicine. There are tremendous volumes of data already in the public domain. For example, a DNA microarray or "gene chip" can quantitate every gene in the genome. This high-throughput genome technology is now widely used in research laboratories and has led to massive volumes of microarray data. One of the repositories tasked with holding these data is the National Center for Biotechnology Information (NCBI) Gene Expression Omnibus (GEO). This United States–based repository currently contains more than 625,000 publicly available microarray datasets. Together with a comparable European repository, there are more than 900,000 microarray datasets in the public domain. At the current pace, the content doubles every 2 years (Butte, 2008).

Commoditization of Data

Data generation has been commoditized, Butte said. He offered the example of Assay Depot, an online marketplace for scientific research services. One can search for anything from assays to animal models and can purchase services from vendors "as easily as finding a song on iTunes." These are laboratories around the world with excess capacity that are ready to do business with "dry bench" researchers, as well as laboratories in need of a specific service or laboratories that find they get faster results, or higher-quality results, by outsourcing these types of services via the Internet than by using the local university facility.

At this point, most of the steps along the translational pipeline can be commoditized, including clinical and molecular measurements, statistical and computational methods, and validation. The step that cannot be commoditized or outsourced, Butte said, is asking good questions. Given all of the public data, what are the new kinds of questions we should be asking? Given this commoditization of data, one no longer needs a wet lab to conduct academic research or launch commercial research ventures. All one needs is a place to formulate questions (and the means to pay for the studies).

Integrative Genomics to Identify Novel Targets

The first example Butte described involves using integrative genomics on public data to find causal factors for complex diseases, factors that can be targets for new drugs. Butte argued that the only way forward for some complex diseases will be to develop algorithms to integrate genetic, genomic, proteomic, preclinical model, and clinical data.

A decade ago, Butte and colleagues conducted a microarray study on type 2 diabetes and identified 187 genes that were differentially expressed in diabetes and non-diabetes muscle tissue (Patti et al., 2003). Now, intersecting those data with the results of 130 similar independent microarray experiments looking at muscle, fat, beta cells, and liver from rat, mouse, and human, Butte sought to identify common genes across all of these tissues and species (Kodama et al., 2012). Most of the genes in the genome were positive in just one of those studies. One gene, which Butte referred to as Gene A, was differently expressed between diabetes and control samples in 78 of the diabetes microarray experiments but, remarkably, had never been pursued for elucidation of the pathophysiology of type 2 diabetes. Further study by Butte and his group showed that Gene A codes for a functioning cell-surface receptor. Another common differentially expressed gene, which he referred to as Gene C, codes for the ligand for that receptor. Subsequent studies in mice (done through collaboration or purchased services, Butte noted) showed that the receptor is upregulated in mice fed a high-fat diet and is expressed on inflammatory cells in adipose tissue. Gene A turns out to be a well-known receptor, and a knockout mouse is available from Jackson Laboratories. Further testing showed that the knockout mouse had increased insulin sensitivity (i.e., does not die from diabetes and fares better than the wild type), which Butte suggested is why this gene was never studied further for diabetes.

Knocking out this receptor now makes this an interesting therapeutic target, Butte said. Because a soluble form of Gene A protein can be detected in the blood, serum from patients was assayed for the diabetes marker, hemoglobin A1c (HbA1c), and Gene A protein. The data show that the lower the level of the receptor, the lower the level of HbA1c. Treatment for 7 days with therapeutic antibody to Gene A protein lowered the blood sugar of mice fed a high-fat diet.

In summary, Butte said, by using publicly available data that anyone can access, a protodrug, an antireceptor antibody, and a serum companion diagnostic have been developed, all in about 18 months. There are also human pathology data, mouse models, and human genetics data. Butte and colleagues have used the same approach for type 1 diabetes, small-cell lung cancer, and other diseases.

Genomic Nosology and Drug or Diagnostic Discovery

In another approach, Butte sought to find every microarray experiment that has looked at normal and disease samples in the same experiment. Many cancer researchers study metastatic versus nonmetastatic disease, but very few studies actually include normal controls. The first challenge was discovering that there were 200 words for "normal" in the repository (e.g., normal, vehicle, wild type, control, time zero, margins).

From the searches, a systematic classification of disease based on similarities in gene expression was assembled. Butte highlighted the fact that colon cancer and colon polyps clustered together based on molecular profiles (as would be expected since certain polyps are associated with cancer); however, cervical cancer was most similar to type 1 autoimmune polyglandular syndrome. In other words, cervical cancer was more similar to a very rare pediatric genetic disease that is not a cancer than it was to another cancer, colon cancer.

Around the same time, the Broad Institute released the Connectivity Map, a repository of genomewide transcriptional expression data from human cell lines treated with more than 1,500 different drugs at varying doses. Matching the disease gene expression data with the drug gene expression data, Butte identified hundreds of correlations and is currently pursuing two: a seizure drug, topiramate, that may be effective for inflammatory bowel disease and an ulcer drug, cimetidine (Tagamet), that may be effective on lung adenocarcinoma (Sirota et al., 2011). Both have shown efficacy in animal models.

Again, Butte stressed, this entire work was done using publicly available data, and he urged investment in building these types of repositories, keeping them updated, and facilitating access to them.

In conclusion, Butte said, bioinformatics is more than just building tools. There are plenty of tools published every month, and the molecular, clinical, and epidemiological data already exist. There are thousands, perhaps tens of thousands, of repositories today. We can identify new diagnostics, therapeutics, and disease mechanisms by integrating datasets. We just need to demonstrate what can be done, he said.

Finally, there is a need for investigators who can imagine the basic questions to ask of these clinical and genomic repositories and are willing to make a career of studying publicly available data. Investigators need to move beyond the mindset that "if it's not your own data you can't trust it." The data are just sitting there, Butte said, waiting for people to use them.

ADAPTING TO DATA-INTENSIVE, DATA-ENABLED BIOMEDICINE

Data represent the fastest-growing resource on Earth, said George Poste, chief scientist for the Complex Adaptive Systems Initiative at Arizona State University. The volume, variety, and speed with which new data are being generated in biomedicine are staggering, and the current computational power may not be sufficient. Data are global and range across multiple users and scales, from the molecular level to the patient in the clinic. The central challenge is how to integrate these data.

Data Production, Analysis, and Utilization in Biomedicine

Poste summarized the overarching themes in meeting the biomedical informatics challenges as the following:

- systems,
- scale, standards, and sharing,

- software, storage, and security,
- sustainability, and
- social issues (changing mindsets and behaviors).

With regard to data production in biomedicine, Poste said, there are more data, but many reported findings have not been validated, and there are issues with replication, suitability for a specified purpose (e.g., regulatory), and authenticity (e.g., information on the Internet). There are more powerful, high-throughput analytic tools, but we deploy them against small sets of samples, resulting in inadequate analytic and statistical rigor. Technology convergence and the creation of multidisciplinary datasets are handicapped by single-specialty silos. There are more participants, locations, and distributed data, but there is a pervasive lack of interoperable exchange formats and standards for data annotation, analysis, and curation. There is also a poor record of sharing.

Data analysis and utilization in biomedicine, Poste said, require more rapid, real-time data access, but data are often trapped in isolated and hierarchical databanks. There is a need for more quantification and precision analytics, but insufficient numbers of personnel are trained for large-scale data analysis. More complexity and uncertainty exist, but there are escalating gaps in institutional and individual cognitive and analytic capabilities to handle it. Finally, the rate of change in data is increasing, as is the rate at which our knowledge and competencies depreciate.

Most of the current approaches to bioinformatics and health care informatics lack the agility and extensibility to meet projected needs, whether in basic or clinical research. We need much more sophisticated approaches for end-to-end system design, Poste said. Systems must meet the needs of a multiplicity of end-user communities without creating new silos. Ours is a data-driven, data-enabled society. Most data are now fundamentally networked, and an increasing fraction of data is digital from the outset. But as datasets become ever larger, they become increasingly unmovable with the existing infrastructure. Sophisticated simulations and meta-analytics can amplify the data streams.

Poste referred to the "fourth paradigm" of scientific discovery espoused by computer scientist Jim Gray, which states that we are now in a period of data-driven knowledge, intelligence, and actionable decisions (following the earlier paradigms of experiment, theory, and simulation). The nature of discovery has moved from hypothesis driven to hypothesis generating, based upon the analysis of large datasets, and explanation involves complex statistical probabilities instead of simplistic, unitary (particularly binary) values.

Having reviewed the gaps and challenges, Poste asked if we are still building systems and infrastructure that merely support the collection of data or are working toward an integrated knowledge ecosystem that supports moving the data from discovery to actionable intelligence that can drive a learning health care enterprise.

Importance of Having the "Right" Data in the System

Poste stressed the importance of pre-analytical variables such as rigorous selection of specimen donors, standardized specimen collection, and annotated health records. Most researchers, however, do not have access to highly standardized, stringently collected, and phenotyped patient samples. He quoted Carolyn Compton, former director of the NIH Office of Biorepositories and Biospecimen Research and now president and CEO of C-Path, who has stated in several venues that "the technological capacity exists to produce low-quality data from low-quality analytes with unprecedented efficiency . . . we now have the ability to get the wrong answers with unprecedented speed." This is a pervasive problem in biomarker identification and validation, which suffers from a "small N" problem that leads to bias and overfitting. It has been suggested that more than 50 percent of the data from academic labs cannot be replicated by industry for new drug target validation and submission to the FDA (Ioannidis and Panagiotou, 2011; Mullard, 2011).

The ability of each individual to have his or her genome sequenced inexpensively will add to the complexity. He said that having this genome information will allow for modulation of gene expression that can be transmitted transgenerationally, altering the epigenome in the progeny. The 95 percent of the genome that is noncoding is also turning out to be profoundly important in regulating the other 5 percent, Poste said.

What is going to represent a complete and accurate analysis of genome sequence, architecture, and regulation, Poste asked, for the purposes of informing regulatory and clinical decisions? He cited a recent publication describing only 88 percent concordance of single-nucleotide variants when the same samples were analyzed on two different sequencing platforms (Lam et al., 2011). The FDA is currently reviewing validation issues for the clinical use of genome sequencing.

Researchers also can access numerous protein–protein interaction and pathway databases, based on the critical assumption that the databases are accurate, he said, citing Schnoes and colleagues (2009), who describe inaccuracies and misannotations in large primary protein databases (including GenBank NR and TeEMBL).

As discussed by Leroy Hood (Chapter 3), mapping the dysregulation of biological networks in disease is a rational foundation for targeted drug discovery. The goal is to target an intervention where the network is being perturbed. However, these are complex, adaptive systems, and a unifocal point intervention in a network will almost certainly be compensated for or have a bypass circuit available. One approach is to try to define network choke points as targets, subverting the alternate compensatory pathways as well. He said a challenging question in cancer drug development is, "At what point does the level of network dysregulation eclipse any feasible approach to achieve a homeostatic reset with drugs?" In this regard, Poste suggested that diagnostic technologies for early detection may be the more prudent option for research investments.

In summary, Poste said that a huge amount of data being put into the public domain is not accurate. Moving forward, Poste listed the need for controlled vocabularies and ontologies; minimal information checklists and open source repositories; algorithms and source code for analytic tools; exchange formats and semantic interoperability; and cross-domain harmonization, integration, migration, and sharing. Ultimately, the only valuable data are validated, actionable data.

Computational Capabilities for Large Datasets

Other disciplines are skilled at handling big datasets, but Poste suggested that insularity makes us reluctant to look at, learn from, and import these approaches into biomedicine.

Most of us, he said, have been trained in "static world" biomedicine that involves conventional collaborations, traditional social and professional preferences and hierarchies, minimum patient input, and a general reluctance to share data. The world we live in, however, is increasingly dynamic. This includes web-based collaborations, fluid populations of diverse participants with many unanticipated productive inputs, the ability to mine huge amounts of public data, open source networks, and extended communities.

Despite this overall movement toward increased access, a 2009 review of the top 500 papers published in the 50 journals that had the highest impact factor found that only 9 percent had deposited the primary raw data into a public database (Alsheikh-Ali et al., 2011). Of the portion of the 500 papers that were covered by a journal or funding agency data access policy, 59 percent were not compliant.

Access to the raw data and computer code is absolutely essential, Poste stressed, and new incentives are needed to encourage people to share data. There is a need for ways to ensure due credit, attribution, and citation of the original dataset when it is used by others. He said the greatest challenge, however, is how to drive molecular medicine and IT-centric capabilities in routine clinical medicine. Designing next-generation health IT systems that will comprehensively capture the genetic, biological, behavioral, social, environmental, and ecological factors relevant to disease risk, progression, and outcomes is extremely challenging. Electronic health records need to be thought of in a dynamic sense, rather than simply a digital version of the original fixed paper format. Most EHRs, however, are not designed to support secondary use of data. A comprehensive clinical data integration system would include, for example, current and planned clinical trials, observational data from the provider as well as patient-reported information, SEER data, mobile health or remote sensor data, and payer datasets.

The final reckoning for actionable data is regulatory science, Poste said. Yet while there are many references to personalized medicine in FDA strategic planning documents, Poste noted that there is scant reference to how the challenges of personalized medicine will be met, including the informatics needs.

We have the capability to create a new health care ecosystem from the convergence of technologies and markets, Poste said (Figure 5-1), but this depends upon cyberinfrastructure for both e-science and e-medicine. He referred participants to the recently released report from the National Science Foundation (NSF, 2012) on cyberinfrastructure needs for 21st century science and engineering. If we do have standardized, validated data, how do we move them? Most academic data remain isolated in laboratories or centers. Contemporary academia does not have the necessary connectivity (e.g., optical networks with 10,000 megabit per second transfer) or the computational capacity to gain access to the data it needs. There is a growing imbalance between the ability of the end-user population to access data and embrace their complexity and the ability (or lack thereof) of institutions to access and analyze large sets of data. Poste suggested that institutions that cannot harness big datasets will suffer "cognitive starvation" and relegation to competitive irrelevance in the scientific and engineering domains.

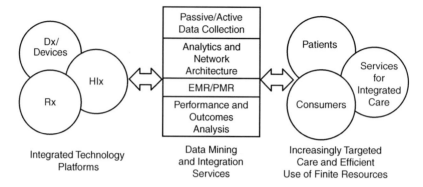

FIGURE 5-1 A new health care ecosystem arising from convergence of technologies and markets.
NOTE: Dx = diagnostics; EMR = electronic medical record; HIx = health information; PMR = personal medical record; Rx = (bio)pharmaceuticals.
SOURCE: Poste presentation (February 28, 2012).

Whether one has access to a high-performance computing center internally or participates with others in a consortium to create a cluster that provides high-performance computing capability, the cloud is a ubiquitous option. There are numerous commercial cloud computing services, and there is no single business model for cloud computing adoption at this stage. Poste noted that although the cloud provides on-demand access to large-scale, economically competitive computing capacity and flexibility, there are concerns about security, reliability, intellectual property, and regulatory compliance.

Moving from Silos to Systems

Moving forward begins with changing minds and changing behaviors to transition from informational silos to integrated systems. Technology is only the enabler, Poste said. We must embrace new organizational structures and must engage and educate multiple constituencies. The health care space will become increasingly decentralized with regard to how data are generated and increasingly centralized for data analytics and decision support. Data flows will increase as patient encounters with the health care system evolve from being episodic to more continuous, real-time monitoring.

In developing a new framework that can adapt to the scale and logistical complexity of modern biomedicine, Poste suggested that research sponsors (e.g., NIH) focus less on single-investigator awards that offer incremental progress and instead seek to fund high-risk and high-reward projects with the potential for radical, disruptive innovation; that a single-discipline career focus be replaced with obligate assembly of diverse expertise for multidimensional engagement; that new study sections with broader expertise, including industry, be assembled; and that siloed datasets be abandoned for large-scale, standardized, interoperable open source databases with professional annotation, analytics, and curation.

Government has a vital role to play, Poste said, in the promulgation of standards, centralized coordination of resources, enforcement of data sharing, and proactive design of regulatory frameworks to address new technologies. Industry plays an important role by participating in pre-competitive private–public partnerships and by taking a proactive role in shaping new transdisciplinary education, training, and employment opportunities.

Ours is a world of massive data, Poste summarized, and to manage these data we need disruptive change and new products, services, and partnership models. He emphasized that moving forward will require *courage* to declare that radical change is needed; *resilience* to combat denial and deflection by entrenched constituencies; *competitiveness and new participants* who drive disruption at the margins or at convergence points (the voice of patients, payers, and new industrial participants will drive e-science and health IT); and *accountability and responsibility*, providing improved return on investment of public and private funding and addressing urgent societal and economic imperatives.

BIG DATA AND DISRUPTIVE INNOVATION: MODELS FOR DEMOCRATIZING CANCER RESEARCH AND CARE

More so than in any other area of health care, cancer research and cancer care are especially overloaded by data, said Jason Hwang, executive director of Health Care at the Innosight Institute. Before the advent of next-generation sequencing techniques, the doubling time of DNA sequencing data was about 19 months, slightly slower than the doubling time of hard-disk storage capacity (about 14 months). After the uptake of new sequencing technologies, however, the doubling time of sequencing data decreased dramatically to around 5 months (Stein, 2010). Sequence data are just one component of biomedical data. Combined with all of the data being generated in the clinic and in research, the volume of biomedical data, especially cancer-related data, is growing exponentially.

As an internist who subsequently earned a master of business administration, Hwang said that many of the problems facing biomedicine are common challenges that other industries have solved or are also trying to solve. The challenges of big data are not unique to health care, and studying the approaches used by industries (e.g., retail, airlines, banking) can be very informative, he said.

Learning from Users of Big Data in Diverse Non-Health Venues

The idea of using big data to make better decisions is not new and predates computing by a number of years, Hwang said. He provided one example of big data before the existence of computers that comes from the U.S. Navy. Matthew Fontaine Maury (1806–1873), referred to as the Pathfinder of the Seas and the Scientist of the Seas, is also considered the father of modern oceanography and naval meteorology. In his time, each ship charted its own course across the ocean, and in general, the experience of any given ship that made it across was not shared. Maury realized that data collected on a voyage (e.g., meteorological data, currents, winds) were trapped in silos (the ship's log) and that these data could be integrated to create optimal routes for any ship on any given day. He created a standardized reporting mechanism that included a reward for any ship captain that submitted his log books along with the maps that Maury had provided. He then compiled these data and revised his maps for the next journey.

Another more recent example that Hwang described involves a group of mathematicians and computer enthusiasts who were dubbed "the gang that beat Las Vegas." Until that time, betting lines and odds were set by individual bookkeepers who made predictions based on the (generally limited) information to which they had access, adjusting their betting lines based on trends and statistics and the bookkeeper's intuition. Members of the computer group realized that if they had access to computing power, they could plug in all of the available data, more than any individual bookkeeper could ever hope to assemble and process, and probably do much better on the odds, Hwang explained. They collected data not just on last week's game results, but on all of the opponent's games, the weather, the latest injury reports, etc. Ultimately, the group fared so well that no one in Las Vegas would take its bets anymore, and a syndicate of people had to be created to place these bets. According to Federal Bureau of Investigation (FBI) records, between 1980 and 1985, the main members of the group amassed close to $14 million in profits (about $20 million to $25 million in today's dollars), with a return on investment of more than 10 percent. Because this number included only members of the core computer group and did not include many other bets placed by family members and friends with whom they shared odds data, the actual profits are likely quadruple that amount. Although they were indicted for other crimes (related to placing bets over the phone), the FBI was never able to charge them with the most serious crime of bookkeeping.

No matter the industry, data abound. It is what we are able to do with the data that is important, Hwang said. Many modern success stories of the use of big data are not particularly representative of their traditional industries, for example, Amazon.com (retailer, bookseller) and Netflix (video distribution). They excel at data collection and use it to drive decisions that improve their business model day after day.

For example, Hwang said that Netflix realized that a video rental service by mail is easily commoditized and has a low barrier to entry and that any number of start-ups could have entered the same space. What Netflix also realized was that it could collect data on people's preferences and start making customized recommendations, making it the service of choice. Two-thirds of video selections made on Netflix are driven by the recommendations its software makes. Amazon collects data on what people decide to purchase, as well as what they clicked on and decided not to purchase, and uses these data to make recommendations of "you may also like. . . ." These data on unchosen clicks (or "data exhaust") that were processed and incorporated into Amazon's decision making are often thrown away by other companies, Hwang noted.

Another big data user, Google, developed its search engine in a way that was very different from anybody else, Hwang said. Google realized that if it gave you a list of ranked search results and you clicked on number four instead of number one, and dozens of other people did that as well, this was an opportunity to improve its search results (e.g., rank that number four result higher next time). Using this data exhaust, Google was able to create the best spell-checkers for nearly every language in the world. Every time someone misspells something, Google will suggest what it thinks they mean, but it gives them the opportunity to say, "No, I meant to spell it that way." If enough people say that is how they intended to spell it, Google takes the opportunity to learn and improve its spell-checker. Google has built its translators in a similar learning fashion. Google is rapidly expanding its translation engines and capabilities in a way that is far cheaper, because it is essentially crowdsourcing its software construction, Hwang explained.

The real impact of big data, Hwang suggested, is that the data will allow better decision making based on computer algorithms, rather than relying upon just one expert's individual opinion (which can vary widely among experts, especially in health care). Data-based algorithms could aid in choosing the most appropriate treatment when there are multiple to choose from, for example. This is not unlike the transformation in banking, Hwang said, where previously a loan officer had to base a decision about people's ability to repay on factors such as the type of clothes they wore and the car they drove, their job and how long they worked there, marital status, and so forth. With better analytics, computerized credit reporting and monitoring services now help make that decision, in many cases replacing the human decision maker. This opens up the door to other opportunities, Hwang said, such as allowing consumers to see the criteria on which their creditworthiness is based and to optimize their credit score in order to get the best loans possible.

Disruptive Innovation

In the ability to use big data there is opportunity to create new economies. If we think of the marketplace as concentric circles, Hwang said, customers who have the most money and the most expertise are at the center. These are the people who are the early adopters of any new product or service in an industry. Moving outward in the rings, the amount of money and expertise diminishes, until the outermost circle represents the people with the least amount of money and the least amount of expertise, who are the last adopters of any product or service.

Using service industries as an example, Hwang explained that solutions have classically been very centralized. That is, if there is a problem that needs to be solved, we go to a source of the solution and pay that source for the expertise to help solve the problem. In essence, technologies have now extracted that expertise from the brain of the expert and embedded it in a piece of software, a tool, or a technology, such that anyone can use it. This commoditizes that expertise and democratizes access to industries by making it convenient and affordable. When booking travel, for example, no longer does one need to always call a travel agent. Most people are capable of making a simple booking using the tools available online. There are sources of decision support to help people make the right decision for their needs. While travel agents are still there to help with more complicated needs, there is choice in the marketplace, granted by technologies that have commoditized travel expertise. This can be observed in many different industries. One can go to an accountant or choose to use TurboTax or some other type of software support that commoditizes the expertise of tax accountants. One can choose to go to a bank teller during banking hours or to an automated teller machine (ATM) whenever one wants.

Convenience and personal empowerment drive the disruption that we see in service industries, and Hwang said that this will be the case for health care as well. Think now of the centralized source not as a travel agent, an accountant, or a real estate agent, but as the local general hospital. Many health care services are either embedded within or revolve around the big general hospital in every local district. In this case, the goal of disruptive innovation is to suggest that the expertise and tasks being done in general hospitals today could be shifted outside such that people do not have to travel to the hospital for care. What services can be provided in an outpatient setting? What tools and technologies could equip a general practitioner to do what only groups of specialists would normally do in the wards of a hospital? Further, what is being done in the outpatient setting that could be delivered in a doctor's office or even a kiosk and could be delivered not just by doctors but by nurse practitioners, pharmacists, physician assistants, and allied health professionals? Ultimately, what can be done in patients' homes and managed by patients themselves? Disruptive innovation is about where health care can exist in a sustainable and affordable fashion in this country, Hwang said.

Big data can help to facilitate the decentralization of our highly centralized and expensive health care structure and help to emphasize prevention and wellness. Hwang listed some of the many different types of data-enabled business models that could help to achieve decentralized health care, including telehealth and e-visits, automated kiosks, home monitoring, wireless health devices, retail and worksite clinics, and others. All of these are enabled by technologies such as telecommunications and precision diagnostics as well as better decision-making tools that are derived from big data (Figure 5-2).

The goal is not to put hospitals and doctors out of business, Hwang stressed; however, health care delivery is a scarce resource that could well be supplemented by this approach. He likened the potential for decentralization in health care to what has happened in the legal world. Simple actions that used to be done by lawyers, such as trademark registration, small business incorporation, simple real estate leases, and legal discovery, for example, fall into a category that economists call "automating the automat-

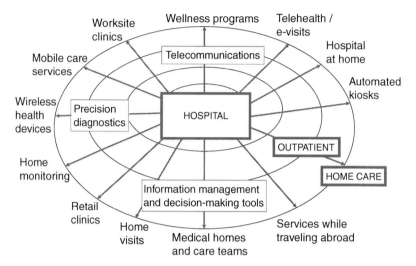

FIGURE 5-2 A new ecosystem of disruptive business models.
SOURCE: Hwang presentation (February 28, 2012).

able." For example, software programs can now assemble documents that used to require hours of work. When software can manage some of the tasks that used to be reserved only for professionals, it frees up the professionals so that they can spend far more time talking to their clients and focusing on higher-value work, where their expertise is really needed.

In summary, Hwang predicted that big data will transform cancer care and research first, because the data deluge in the field outpaces anything else in health care. Building EHRs and other data repositories is just the beginning; the truly sustainable value will be provided by enterprises capable of extracting wisdom from the data. The ultimate goal, he said, is to use big data to create the tools that will commoditize expertise and make care more accessible to more people.

Democratizing Big Data Informatics for Cancer and Other Therapeutic Areas

Kris Joshi, global vice president of health care for Oracle, expanded on the concept of democratization of informatics. With so many sources of data currently or soon to be available (e.g., the anticipated $100 genome, mobile health devices, imaging), the challenge is providing people with tools that are affordable, readily available, and easily manageable so they can derive value from the data. Patients are interested in a value-based health system that consistently delivers new therapies and better care at a cost they can afford, but they do not want affordability at the expense of innovation, Joshi said. Similarly, patients want privacy protection, but they understand that collaboration across the life sciences and health care is necessary to achieve this innovation, and they do not want collaboration to be stopped under the guise of privacy protection.

Joshi likened informatics to an iceberg. The small tip that is visible is the data analysis and presentation that everyone is interested in doing. The challenge is the rest of the iceberg lurking below the surface—the data acquisition from myriad complex clinical, financial, administrative, and research source systems and the attendant cleansing, integration, and warehousing of these data. This is almost always underappreciated in terms of the magnitude of the work involved, Joshi said.

Informatics done right can transform health systems to a point where the insights coming out of EHR data can be translated within the institution into improved processes and procedures that reflect the best knowledge, not from 10 years ago but from 2 weeks ago, because that knowledge was incorporated in a learning health care workflow (Figure 5-3). A closed-loop learning health care system empowers clinicians and nurses who can look at the data and effect change. However, current health IT systems do not have the capability to support this.

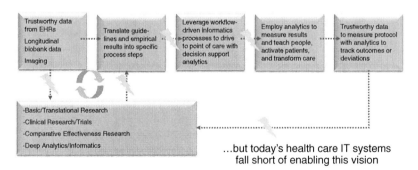

FIGURE 5-3 Learning health care paradigm supported by robust, interoperable informatics.

NOT: EHR = electronic medical record.
SOURCE: Joshi presentation February 28, 2012. Reprinted with permission from Kris Joshi and Brett Davis.

The fundamental problem is turning the growing mass of data into transformational insights. Because biases in the data can lead different individuals to reach different conclusions, transparency in how one derived the insight from the data is critical, Joshi stressed. These challenges are general informatics problems (i.e., not specific to cancer or even specific to research), and they should be solved like general informatics problems, Joshi said. Also, as noted by others, much can be learned from other industries. He added that in trying to solve one problem, you often find that some of the solutions also solve another problem elsewhere in the health care ecosystem (e.g., addressing a research informatics issue also ends up solving a payer issue).

Many decisions are now made using analytics, which must be reproducible if one is to be able to justify the decision. Analytics, Joshi said, is a niche industry where only those who know how to deal with the data can derive value from it, and this keeps analytics from being a highly used tool.

One ongoing challenge in analytics has been integrating and normalizing data from the different source systems (e.g., clinical, financial, administrative, research). A lot of data quality problems start at this point, Joshi noted. The informatics requirements for data integration, validation, and normalization are not trivial and require an enterprise approach. However, once a core enterprise analytics platform is in place, numerous applications can be developed that allow researchers, clinicians, administrators, and others to analyze those high-quality data. A common infrastructure can also support multiple secondary uses of data and thereby lower costs. For example, data can be used for clinical trial optimization, decreasing time lines and enhancing efficiency and accuracy. Joshi suggested that in addition to thinking about secondary uses of data, we should consider secondary uses of IT infrastructure as another way to reduce overall costs. Specifically, creating an entire system focused on cancer runs the risk of spending too much time, effort, and money; not focusing on innovation; and most likely duplicating existing systems to some extent.

In closing, Joshi mentioned one example of the regional initiatives that are gearing up to enable collaboration across the health care ecosystem: the Partnership to Advance Clinical electronic Research (PACeR) initiative, which is a public–private partnership between New York State hospitals and life sciences companies.

Consumers as Disruptive Innovators

The Patient Protection and Affordable Care Act (ACA) put in place incentives for coordination of care and for innovation around patient engagement, explained Farzad Mostashari, national coordinator for health information technology in the Office of the National Coordinator for Health Information Technology (ONC). Insurers no longer want to pay for care as piecework, he said. Per the ACA, if hospitals can provide care for Medicare patients that is more coordinated, they can share in any resulting savings.

Mostashari listed three elements that will aid in the successful coordination of care: (1) the technology infrastructure for care coordination exists, (2) there is a strong business case for care coordination and patient engagement, and (3) there is movement toward the democratization of information and information tools. The consumer is the ultimate disrupter here, he said.

As a case example, Mostashari offered his thoughts on some of the reasons Google Health failed. While certain elements are specific to Google, others are more generalizable, and we can learn from them. First, people had to spend hours typing in their own information. Per HIPAA, patients have a right to get a copy of their own medical information (and certain legislative provisions may require that it be provided electronically and within a specified time period). It is legally possible for people to get access to their own records, but it should also be easy to do. People are often uncomfortable asking for their records, worrying that asking is in some way challenging the doctor, Mostashari added. This attitude needs to change, he said. Knowing your information is part of what being a good patient is about.

Another problem with Google Health, Mostashari said, was that once people typed all of their information in, they could not do much more with it except read or print it. People want to be able to find a clinical trial, learn what the side effects of their medications are, get a second opinion, see their images, share their data, or keep abreast of the latest research on their cancer. They want to find resources and find other people like themselves.

The progress in health IT for doctors and hospitals is exciting, Mostashari said, but what is more exciting is the disruptive possibilities of consumers and their caregivers as the nexus where information comes together and is used to generate new knowledge.

THE EHR AND CANCER RESEARCH AND CARE

Enhancing Uptake of EHRs

Mostashari said that when he joined ONC in 2009, about 10 percent of hospitals and 20 percent of primary care providers used a basic EHR system. The Health Information Technology for Economic and Clinical Health Act (HITECH) of 2009 put in place financial incentives for doctors and hospitals to adopt and meaningfully use EHRs and created some of the digital infrastructure to help small practices. By 2011, 37 percent of hospitals were using an EHR system. Mostashari anticipated that by 2013, it would be more than 50 percent.

The EHR is not just an office system, he said. ONC has developed interoperability standards to facilitate sharing and has a program to certify EHR systems that conform to these standards. Per the standards, information on clinical care, medications, procedures, and other data will be in a standard XML format with tags to tell users what the data elements are and where they go. Data will be shared when patients transition from care setting to care setting. Data will also be shared with the patient, because this is one of the requirements for meaningful use of an EHR, Mostashari noted.

The EpicCare System as a Model for the Uses of EHRs in Cancer Research and Care

Sam Butler, a physician and member of the clinical informatics team at software developer Epic, described the features of the EpicCare system as a model for the uses of EHRs in cancer research and care. He estimates that EpicCare has been used for somewhere between 108 million and 142 million patients in the United States, across 270 health care clients. An available add-on module to the main EHR is Beacon, Epic's oncology information system. Currently, Butler explained, Beacon is primarily for chemotherapy management. Functions include staging, problem lists, protocols, treatment planning, review and release, pharmacy verification, electronic medication administration record (eMAR), flow sheets, and reporting. Of the 270 current EpicCare EHR users, 140 of them are actively installing Beacon.

The system is extensible, and it is easy for an institution to add information to a set of problems. The model system includes 250 protocols, both standardized regimens and research protocols. These are not meant to be a review of the literature, Butler noted, but are representative protocols using standard protocol language to serve as starting points. Customers are required to review the protocols, validate them, and make them their own protocols. A protocol can be adapted as a treatment plan for a particular patient. Once a treatment plan is created, nurses review the information when a patient arrives, and the nurse or pharmacist releases the orders, which then go through a process of pharmacy verification. Administration of treatment is instantly documented in the eMAR, often by using bar coding. Everything is captured in the flow sheet, which informs and supports physician decision making regarding the next round of treatment. Then the cycle of treatment plan, pharmacy verification, eMAR documentation, and flow sheet begins again. Beacon can also capture discrete data such as reasons for changing a treatment plan or discontinuing it.

This cyclical system works well in a large institution where the oncologists, pharmacists, and nurses all are in the same organization. However, if the physicians are in their community practice and they have another EHR, or another program to create their treatment plan, there is no standard to communicate that treatment plan to a hospital, infusion center, or pharmacist with a different system.

Application and workbench data are exported nightly or more frequently and deposited into a reporting database that is relational and that can be accessed by analytic tools. The data can also be combined with other data warehouses or biorepositories in other systems. The database can be used to create custom data marts that are customer developed and owned.

In the future, the system will allow more patient-entered data. Epic is working on ways to engage patients, such as sending out surveys, aggregating the data that are reported, and displaying that information in graphs and reports to help patients make an informed decision about their treatment by showing them what other patients have experienced. The challenge, Butler noted, will be getting enough patient data to make those graphs meaningful and significant. Epic is also working on incorporating genomics and adding the ability to document the care a patient received before entering this system, for a complete oncological history.

Butler noted several challenges in moving forward, including encouraging physicians to see the value of using an EHR (he said physicians are very concerned that using an EHR is going to slow them down), interoperability, and management of big datasets.

CANCER CENTER–BASED NETWORKS FOR HEALTH RESEARCH INFORMATION EXCHANGE

Following on his discussion of the informatics challenges facing cancer centers (Chapter 2), William Dalton, of the Moffitt Cancer Center, offered an aspirational model for a research and health care information exchange network that would allow many different partners and stakeholders to participate, contribute, and benefit (Figure 5-4). Expanding on the research information exchange he described earlier (see Figure 2-3), the data warehouse would become a federated network information system.

Personalized Cancer Care

The development of personalized cancer care relies on the efforts of many people contributing to the continuous cycle of discovery, translation, and delivery of health care. Data networks allow for the discovery of associations between specific molecular profiles and clinical information from individual patients, leading to new knowledge that can be translated into more personalized cancer care.

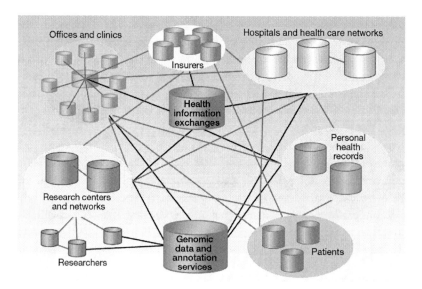

FIGURE 5-4 Designing a new federated research and health care network model.
SOURCE: Dalton et al., 2010. Reprinted with permission from the American Association for Cancer Research.

One approach to facilitate personalized care is to ask patients to participate as partners in the care journey. As an example, Dalton described the Moffitt "Total Cancer Care Protocol." This IRB-approved observational study protocol includes three critical questions for the patient:

1. Can we follow you throughout your lifetime? (With the goal of entering any health care data into a central data warehouse)
2. Can we study your tumor using molecular technology? (With the goal of entering genetic and genomic data into a central data warehouse)
3. Can we recontact you? (For purposes of sharing information that might be of importance to you, such as a clinical trial designed for patients like you)

As part of a public–private partnership with Merck, the protocol is currently open in a consortium of 18 sites in 10 states, all using the same protocol and consent and following standard operating procedures for tumor collection and data aggregation, and many using the same central IRB. Now finishing its sixth year, more than 85,000 people have been enrolled to date. More than 32,000 tumors have been collected, all clinically annotated according to standard operating procedures, and almost half have been profiled.

Dalton noted that in its early stages, the database was more of a repository than a warehouse, with some of the queries taking weeks, if not months, and Moffitt sought expert assistance from Oracle, TransMed, and Deloitte. Through this strategic partnership, an integrated health research information platform was developed that creates the real-time relationships and associations from disparate data sources that are needed to create new knowledge for improved patient treatments, outcomes, and prevention. Critical to this endeavor was harmonization of the data through creation of a data dictionary. In addition to defined elements, the dictionary also incorporated a means of measuring the quality and veracity of the data. Because patient information resides in many sources, often with different identification numbers, the first challenge was to create a means of cohort identity. Harmonization of the data takes place in the data factory before the data are placed in a warehouse, where they can then be queried for different uses by different partners and stakeholders. The data warehouse is a robust, scalable dataset of oncology patients, Dalton said, and queries are done in real time.

As one example, Dalton described how the data warehouse could be queried for cohort identification. One could, for example, query for females diagnosed and/or treated at Moffitt between 2005 and 2009 with breast cancer, with the histology of infiltrating ductal carcinoma, not otherwise specified, who were stages III to IV at diagnosis and who were estrogen receptor positive, with a documented family history of breast cancer. Out of more than 212,000 female patients in the database, the successive real-time queries identified a cohort of 25. In a second example, Dalton demonstrated how queries could identify patients meeting select clinical trial criteria who were eligible and available at a particular consortium site and who also had banked tissue samples that could be assayed.

Proposed Federated Data Model

It is one thing to be able to do health research information exchange at a single institution or within a defined consortium, but it is quite another, Dalton said, to manage this on a national scale. He proposed a national health and research information exchange, incorporating regional "hub and spoke" platforms, with cancer centers as the hub and their individual colleagues within the community contributing data and having access to those data.

This federated framework could facilitate many aspects of cancer research, including basic science, translational research, drug discovery and development, clinical trials, companion diagnostics, comparative effectiveness and outcomes research, postmarketing surveillance, and others. The goal, as with the other models discussed earlier, is a rapid-learning information system. Each patient added iteratively improves the learning process.

In summary, Dalton said that the guiding principles for developing cancer center collaboration are inclusiveness, accessibility of data (especially real-time access through a research information exchange), and public–private partnerships to achieve long-term sustainability.

OTHER MODELS AND PATHWAYS

During the discussion, panelists offered additional comments on pathways forward and other examples of instructive models in other domains.

Patients Helping Patients

Brandon Hayes-Lattin, cancer survivor, cancer researcher, and senior medical adviser for the Lance Armstrong Foundation, said that the foundation's Share Your Story campaign has transformed cancer survivorship through individual patients posting personal stories so that others might be helped by them. Along these same lines, he supported developing tools where patients could contribute their clinical data to a shared resource and also access aggregated clinical data to guide their personal decision making. He noted that the Livestrong constituency was surveyed regarding sharing their data, and 87 percent of the 8,500 respondents agreed that researchers should have the ability to review their information as long as it is not directly linked to them. Further, 71 percent felt that their data was safer when stored electronically than on paper.

Patients are looking for a range of things, Hayes-Lattin said. They want to trust their physician, but they want to double-check, too. Getting a second opinion requires their raw data, not just the interpretations. Patients also say that they want to be able to find resources. There are a lot of resources available for cancer patients, but it can be hard to find them, he said. It is important for patients to be able to put their situation into context in the larger world of cancer, to learn from the experiences of others.

Bradford Hesse, chief of the NCI Health Communication and Informatics Research Branch, added that a significant portion of traffic to government health websites such as NCI or the Centers for Disease Control and Prevention (CDC) involves patients. Patients are engaged and activated, and they need to have a health system that is prepared to help them. He also referred to the SHARP initiatives (Strategic HIT Advanced Resource Projects), some of which focus on the security and privacy of health IT.

Providing a Substrate for Innovation

Hwang mentioned the role of government in creating a substrate for innovation in the private sector. For example, no private-sector company or start-up was likely going to invent the Internet, but a government agency with the will and the resources did create such a network and opened it up to the private sector for use, essentially launching a new economy. Another example was the launch of global positioning system (GPS) satellites and allowing the private sector to use those data to generate whatever products and services it could imagine. Most companies would not try to launch their own satellites, but many have created innovative products using the data. Poste added that the Internet predecessor, Advanced Research Projects Agency Network (ARPANET), and GPS technology were both products of the military sector. A primary factor driving military technology is a perception of an existential threat. There are similar threats in biomedicine, Poste said, including the economics and viability of the health care system at large and the threat at the level of the individual facing a terrible disease.

In these and other instructive precedents, government has taken the lead in recognizing the threat, recognizing the need for a coherent systems-based approach, and allowing the mobilization of the creativity community (i.e., innovation from the bottom up). Poste argued that what is needed is a combination of national leadership, the courage to acknowledge that much of the system is broken, and the willingness to allow individual, bottom-up contribution and participation in the larger infrastructure.

Mining Data to Assess the Quality of Cancer Care

Allen Lichter, chief executive officer of the American Society of Clinical Oncology (ASCO), noted that ASCO is interested in informatics from a quality-of-care perspective. Quality monitoring is especially important in oncology. As mentioned earlier, most cancer patients are treated in community settings where the vast majority of oncologists are generalists. In addition, diagnostic and therapeutic options are increasing rapidly, and physicians need to make sure that they are up-to-date.

The ASCO Quality Oncology Practice Initiative (QOPI) was designed to monitor the quality of cancer care and has been in place for about 10 years. One concern, Lichter said, is that it assesses quality retrospectively (reviewing cases from 6 months or more prior), uses sample cases, has a limited number of measures, and is manual (taking close to an hour per chart). ASCO is looking to evolve this into a real-time electronic system, reviewing consecutive cases, monitoring the full spectrum of care, and providing decision support.

Fostering Sharing

Butler noted that researchers make their living from their data and they are understandably hesitant to give it up. However, over the course of the workshop there was wide support for the concept that the data should be used to benefit society and should be made available for broad use. Butler suggested starting with data sharing efforts for just a few diagnoses. For example, in pediatric gastroenterology, 30 institutions provide all of their data on inflammatory bowel disease patients to one institution that then aggregates the anonymized data. They did not try to start too big. He added that the United Network for Organ Sharing (UNOS) has done the same with transplant data.

Murphy offered pediatric oncology as a model for collaborating. The field of pediatric oncology has a long history of collecting data and using the information in a virtuous cycle to inform and improve the next generation of care. The field is less competitive and more geared toward sharing.

Education, Training, and Funding

Mia Levy, director of cancer clinical informatics at the Vanderbilt-Ingram Cancer Center, said that there is a real need for more people who are computationally oriented in medical schools. There is also a need for career paths and leadership positions for people who are trained in both medicine and informatics. In funding these researchers, Levy said that review committees need to be receptive to the potential of informatics and the value of observational data.

If Data Are Available, Users Will Come

Levy referred to how Butte and others have made use of publicly available data repositories of cancer information. If data are available, people will start using them for a variety of purposes. To facilitate more use of the data sources that are already available, she said there has to be increased accessibility, more sharing of data, and an invitation to the broader informatics community to come to the table and start working on problems that are important to cancer.

REFERENCES

Alsheikh-Ali, A. A., W. Qureshi, M. H. Al-Mallah, and J. P. Ioannidis. 2011. Public availability of published research data in high-impact journals. *PLoS ONE* 6(9):e24357.

Butte, A. J. 2008. Translational bioinformatics: Coming of age. *Journal of the American Medical Informatics Association* 15(6):709-714.

Dalton, W. S., D. M. Sullivan, T. J. Yeatman, and D. A. Fenstermacher. 2010. The 2010 Health Care Reform Act: A potential opportunity to advance cancer research by taking cancer personally. *Clinical Cancer Research* 16(24):5987-5996.

Ioannidis, J. P., and O. A. Panagiotou. 2011. Comparison of effect sizes associated with biomarkers reported in highly cited individual articles and in subsequent meta-analyses. *Journal of the American Medical Association* 305(21):2200-2210.

Kodama, K., M. Horikoshi, K. Toda, S. Yamada, K. Hara, J. Irie, M. Sirota, A. A. Morgan, R. Chen, H. Ohtsu, S. Maeda, T. Kadowaki, and A. J. Butte. 2012. Expression-based genome-wide association study links the receptor CD44 in adipose tissue with type 2 diabetes. *Proceedings of the National Academy of Sciences* 109(18):7049-7054.

Lam, H. Y., M. J. Clark, R. Chen, R. Chen, G. Natsoulis, M. O'Huallachain, F. E. Dewey, L. Habegger, E. A. Ashley, M. B. Gerstein, A. J. Butte, H. P. Ji, and M. Snyder. 2011. Performance comparison of whole-genome sequencing platforms. *Nature Biotechnology* 30(1):78-82.

Mullard, A. 2011. Reliability of "new drug target" claims called into question. *Nature Reviews Drug Discovery* 10(9):643-644.

NSF (National Science Foundation). 2012. *Advanced computing infrastructure: Vision and strategic plan.* NSF Document nsf12051. http://www.nsf.gov/pubs/2012/nsf12051/nsf12051.pdf (accessed April 27, 2012).

Patti, M. E., A. J. Butte, S. Crunkhorn, K. Cusi, R. Berria, S. Kashyap, Y. Miyazaki, I. Kohane, M. Costello, R. Saccone, E. J. Landaker, A. B. Goldfine, E. Mun, R. DeFronzo, J. Finlayson, C. R. Kahn, and L. J. Mandarino. 2003. Coordinated reduction of genes of oxidative metabolism in humans with insulin resistance and diabetes: Potential role of PGC1 and NRF1. *Proceedings of the National Academy of Sciences* 100(14):8466-8471.

Schnoes, A. M., S. D. Brown, I. Dodevski, and P. C. Babbitt. 2009. Annotation error in public databases: Misannotation of molecular function in enzyme superfamilies. *PLoS Computational Biology* 5(12):e1000605.

Sirota, M., J. T. Dudley, J. Kim, A. P. Chiang, A. A. Morgan, A. Sweet-Cordero, J. Sage, and A. J. Butte. 2011. Discovery and preclinical validation of drug indications using compendia of public gene expression data. *Science Translational Medicine* 3(96):96ra77.

Stein, L. D. 2010. The case for cloud computing in genome informatics. *Genome Biology* 11(5):207.

6

Proposal for a Coalition of All Stakeholders

Marcia Kean, chair of strategic initiatives at Feinstein Kean Healthcare, presented a proposal for a broad stakeholder coalition as one pathway for addressing the informatics needs of the cancer research community. Kean noted that the views expressed by many of the workshop presenters regarding the needs, key elements, and general vision for cancer informatics were compatible with the proposed coalition.

In considering a path forward, Kean said it was important to leverage the successes of previous models of collaboration, exploit existing assets and capabilities, and play to the strengths and needs of all the different constituencies in biomedicine as well as in other industries and communities.

ACHIEVING DATA LIQUIDITY IN THE CANCER COMMUNITY

The proposed coalition was envisioned by Kean as a nonprofit membership organization comprising all stakeholders in the cancer community and beyond, who are deeply committed to actualizing a common vision of data liquidity to achieve personalized cancer care and a rapid-learning health care system. "Data liquidity" refers to the rapid, seamless, secure exchange of useful, standards-based information among authorized individual and institutional senders and recipients. Kean suggested that "rapid" would ideally be real time.

Kean referred participants to several exemplars of data exchange (Cancer Genome Atlas; Biomedical Research Integrated Domain Group,

BRIDG; I-SPY 2 Trial) and noted that the common denominators are that they are all standards-based, manage multidimensional data, and link care and research (i.e., they address the problem of data liquidity). These, and some of the other examples discussed during the workshop, remain isolated efforts, and Kean said that no one is tasked with or responsible for linking them into a national system.

Many of the hurdles to achieving data liquidity were highlighted throughout the workshop (e.g., appropriate sampling; high-quality, validated data; privacy; data ownership; intellectual property; IT infrastructure). If these challenges can be met, the opportunities for personalized cancer medicine and a rapid-learning health care system will abound. Kean suggested that data liquidity could also increase the "velocity of knowledge"—that is, moving from data to information to insights to knowledge to wisdom will happen much faster. This is apparent in other industries, for example, the financial industry.

Principles

Kean outlined the proposed coalition principles (Box 6-1), reiterating that they are open for further discussion. She emphasized that while the proposal calls for open technology frameworks, this does not in any way mean that the commercial IT sector will not play an important role.

Operational Strategy and Activities

As proposed, Kean said that the coalition could deliver rapid, seamless data exchange that would be facilitated by interoperability; driven by just-in-time standards; implemented in small-scale capabilities that are open at the interfaces; and developed incrementally and iteratively to address specific and immediate needs. At the same time, the coalition would be thinking about integrating and coordinating in a systematic way, so that over time these capabilities roll up into a national system.

Kean briefly listed a broad range of activities the coalition could undertake. The coalition could convene; advocate; mobilize participation; serve as an honest broker; select and apply standards and catalyze standards development where none exist; provide consulting and project management services via contracts to members; catalyze the building of capabilities that serve immediate needs via contracts to members or others; leverage success-

> **BOX 6-1**
> **Proposed Coalition Principles**
>
> - Research and clinical care can benefit from collection and analysis of all relevant (and potentially relevant) information, recorded in standards-based formats and curated through appropriate governance structures.
> - Biomedical innovation and achievement of personalized cancer care can be accelerated and improved by facilitating connectivity and seamless data exchange among research and care collaborators.
> - Open IT frameworks—defining standards by which technology components can interoperate—provide such capability through open interfaces, enabling researchers to seamlessly capture, aggregate, integrate, analyze, interpret, and transmit data.
> - Progress toward a connected biomedical community that benefits all health care stakeholders can best be implemented in a pre-competitive setting, where all participants are free to contribute and partake of components.
> - Open technology frameworks—which can facilitate the interface between open source and/or commercial components—must be shared freely.
>
> SOURCE: Kean presentation (February 28, 2012).

ful models of research-enhancing data exchange; act as a guide to advance projects through to completion; and coordinate and integrate capabilities leading up to a national system.

Coalition Governance, Funding, and Sustainability

Kean proposed developing the coalition as a nonprofit organization that would preserve the honest broker role, perhaps as a 501(c)(6) organization, comparable in function to a chamber of commerce. A board of directors would be assembled, with representatives from multiple constituencies. Kean listed several potential mechanisms for funding and sustainability, including membership fees (on a sliding scale), consulting fees, project management fees, foundation grants, and government support.

Working Toward a National System

In working toward a national system of data liquidity, Kean explained, coalition members would be making a commitment of time and resources and would be vested in the success of the resulting capabilities. Each capability would address a specific problem of importance to the user, and once delivered, the capability would be shared. In addition, the coalition would consistently seek to integrate and promulgate the capabilities.

The coalition would be a differentiated, hybrid model in a number of ways, Kean said. It would have the benefit of data exchange through open interfaces while commercial IT companies could be remunerated for their proprietary products or services. It would be a test bed for the capabilities necessary for interoperability. As an open forum, it would seek members from all constituencies; it is not intended to compete with any standard-setting body, but to work adjacent to them and benefit from their work. Importantly, Kean said, the coalition would help ensure that capabilities are not lost as one-off models but rather that they contribute to the national capability.

The coalition would also be different from other efforts, Kean said, in that it would not be a data aggregator or a database; it would not be for the benefit of one single community; it would not be owned or led by the government; it would not undermine proprietary software systems; and it would not be a collection of universal standards. It would also not force data sharing where this is not desired, she added.

A host of potential benefits would accrue from the successful launch and implementation of such a coalition, Kean concluded. In addition to addressing many or even most of the challenges discussed at the workshop, the activities of a successful stakeholder coalition could accelerate studies and advance new approaches to evidence generation and, ultimately, achieve benefits for all constituencies.

In closing, Kean invited participants' feedback on the proposed coalition.

7

Transforming Cancer Informatics: From Silos to Systems

A recurring topic throughout the workshop was the need for change: changing the attitudes, behavior, and culture surrounding the sharing of data and embracing solutions, particularly disruptive solutions, that will drive those changes, according to Sharon Murphy of the IOM. The opportunity is obvious, she said, and society is losing the value of all the data that have been generated by companies, academics, NIH, and others as long as the data are just sitting there. Participants discussed the need to move from silos full of information to integrated systems that provide actionable knowledge to advance cancer care. Scientific and clinical discoveries can be realized much more rapidly with this type of systems infrastructure in place than without, said Lawrence Shulman of Dana-Farber, adding that every year that an important discovery is delayed, thousands of patients die.

Amy Abernethy, associate professor of medicine in the Division of Medical Oncology at the Duke University School of Medicine, summarized the four main themes of discussion throughout the workshop.

Main Workshop Themes Identified by Amy Abernethy

1. **Embrace cancer informatics.** Cancer informatics provides opportunities to do the following:
   - improve the efficiency of the discovery engine;
   - bridge the gap between discovery and health;
   - reduce the risk of losing valuable data assets; and
   - share lessons learned in cancer research so they can be leveraged in cancer care and other medical disciplines.

2. **Embrace solutions.** Embrace complexity and find solutions to address the following issues:
   - data availability, integration, and exchange;
   - democratization of information;
   - technical hurdles;
   - interoperability;
   - governance;
   - value and appropriate use of experimental and observational data;
   - validation and quality;
   - workforce;
   - analytics and methods development;
   - visualization and representation of big datasets; and
   - cyberinfrastructure.

3. **Establish an ecosystem of partners,** including, but not limited to, the following:
   - patients, consumers, advocates;
   - cancer centers, physicians;
   - biomedical research;
   - clinical researchers, quantitative scientists, basic scientists, outcomes researchers; in industry, academia, and government;
   - cancer clinical trials cooperative groups;
   - information technology developers and providers;
   - payers, administrators; and
   - federal agencies.

4. **Generate trust.** Earning the trust of patients, providers, researchers, and society in general is the core underlying issue for the following concerns:
   - data privacy and security;
   - accountability; and
   - data ownership.

A FRAMEWORK FOR ACTION

As a starting point for moving forward, a proposal for a coalition of all stakeholders was introduced during the workshop and participants were urged to provide feedback (see Chapter 6). Abernethy reiterated the main objectives of the proposed coalition as outlined by Marcia Kean of Feinstein Kean Healthcare:

- Catalyze and help nurture a community to develop and make available, pre-competitively, an open digital framework for biomedicine.
- Ensure that the open digital framework stays current with all technological advances.
- Ensure that all biomedical organizations have access to the open digital framework, so that they can achieve their goals for improved patient care and more productive research.
- Help to support a flourishing ecosystem of biomedical organizations that can fuel each other's activities through frictionless flow of data.
- Serve as a test bed for the digital infrastructure.

Changing Minds, Changing Behaviors

As suggested by George Poste (Chapter 5), embracing the complexity of cancer informatics and taking action to drive change will require the courage to acknowledge both the challenges and the need for radical change; the resilience to continue forward in the face of entrenched constituencies; competitiveness and new participants (including consumers) who coordinate and collaborate to generate disruptive change; and accountability and responsibility.

The first step in taking action, Abernethy summarized, is to come together as partners and plan how to move cancer informatics forward (Figure 7-1). Public–private partnerships are essential, she said, as is investing in the data and the cyberinfrastructure. Strategies should leverage the models and successes of other disciplines and industries and should facilitate activities that will contribute to the development of the end-to-end infrastructure system (e.g., just-in-time standards, public databases, EHRs, analytic methods, large-scale standardized protocols and procedures, reuse of data and IT infrastructure, data dictionaries, metadata, validation, and security solutions). Tools should be built with the users and use cases in mind (a bottom-up strategy). Moving forward will also require training, education,

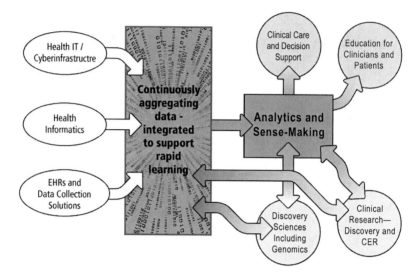

FIGURE 7-1 Hypothetical framework highlighting key elements of an end-to-end cancer informatics system.
NOTE: CER = comparative effectiveness research, EHR = electronic health record, IT = information technology.
SOURCE: Abernethy presentation (February 28, 2012).

and career development to build a workforce that can interface seamlessly across biomedicine, computation, and informatics, she noted.

Apparent throughout the discussion of the gaps, challenges, and potential solutions for cancer informatics was the overarching theme that data should be used for the benefit of society. Data are accumulating fast. "We have the opportunity to harness these data or let them pass us by," Abernethy concluded, and she encouraged participants to "be a part of the plan."

Acronyms

ACA   Patient Protection and Affordable Care Act
ACOSOG   American College of Surgeons Oncology Group
ACRIN   American College of Radiology Imaging Network
AHRQ   Agency for Healthcare Research and Quality
AIM   Annotation and Image Markup
ARPANET   Advanced Research Projects Agency Network
ARRA   American Recovery and Reinvestment Act
ASCO   American Society of Clinical Oncology
ATM   automated teller machine

BRIDG   Biomedical Research Integrated Domain Group

caBIG®   Cancer Biomedical Informatics Grid
CALGB   Cancer and Leukemia Group B
CARE   Comprehensive Accrual REsource
CDC   Centers for Disease Control and Prevention
CER   comparative effectiveness research
CTEP   Cancer Therapy and Evaluation Program
CTMS   clinical trial management system
CTSA   Clinical Translational Science Award
CTSU   Cancer Trials Support Unit

DNA	deoxyribonucleic acid
ECOG	Eastern Cooperative Oncology Group
EHR	electronic health record
ELISA	enzyme-linked immunosorbent assay
eMAR	electronic medication administration record
ER	estrogen receptor
FBI	Federal Bureau of Investigation
FDA	Food and Drug Administration
GCP	Good Clinical Practice
GEO	Gene Expression Omnibus
GPS	global positioning system
HbA1c	hemoglobin A1c
HER2	human epidermal growth factor receptor 2
HHS	U.S. Department of Health and Human Services
HIPAA	Health Insurance Portability and Accountability Act
HITECH	Health Information Technology for Economic and Clinical Health Act
i2b2	Informatics for Integrating Biology and the Bedside
IOM	Institute of Medicine
iPS cells	induced pluripotent stem cells
IRB	institutional review board
IT	information technology
NCBI	National Center for Biotechnology Information
NCCN	National Comprehensive Cancer Network
NCCTG	North Central Cancer Treatment Group
NCI	National Cancer Institute
NHD	Optum Natural History of Disease
NIH	National Institutes of Health
NIMH	National Institute of Mental Health
NSABP	National Surgical Adjuvant Breast and Bowel Project
NSF	National Science Foundation
OCRe	Ontology of Clinical Research

ONC	Office of the National Coordinator for Health Information Technology
QOPI	Quality Oncology Practice Initiative
P4	predictive, preventive, personalized, and participatory
PACeR	Partnership to Advance Clinical electronic Research
PCAST	President's Council of Advisors on Science and Technology
PCORI	Patient-Centered Outcomes Research Institute
RCT	randomized, controlled trial
REDCap	Research Electronic Data Capture
RNA	ribonucleic acid
RTOG	Radiation Therapy Oncology Group
SEER	Surveillance, Epidemiology, and End Results Program
SHARP	Strategic HIT Advanced Resource Projects
siRNA	small interfering RNA
SPARKS	Synergistic Patient and Research Knowledge Systems
SRM	selected reaction monitoring
SWOG	formerly the Southwest Oncology Group
TCGA	The Cancer Genome Atlas
TGen	Translational Genomics Research Institute
UNOS	United Network for Organ Sharing

Appendix A

Workshop Agenda

**INFORMATICS NEEDS AND CHALLENGES
IN CANCER RESEARCH**

February 27 and 28, 2012
The Keck Center of the National Academies
500 Fifth Street, NW—Room 100
Washington, DC 20001

STATEMENT OF TASK

An ad hoc committee will plan and conduct a public workshop whose agenda will examine the informatics needs and challenges for 21st century biomedical research, with a focus on the spectrum of cancer research, ranging from basic science to clinical, comparative effectiveness, and health services delivery research. The workshop, which will feature invited presentations and discussion, will address such topics as

- Design, development, and integration of informatics in cancer research;
- Standards for cancer informatics systems;
- Interoperability and harmonization;
- Infrastructure needs for research;
- Data annotation and curation of multiple complex datasets;

- Methods for data use and representation;
- Implications of implementing effective informatics tools for research; and
- Sustainability, governance, policy, and trust.

Workshop sessions will also include some discussion about how to move beyond the reported shortcomings of the National Cancer Institute's (NCI's) Cancer Biomedical Informatics Grid (caBIG).

The workshop may incorporate illustrative "use cases" reflecting common research applications that rely on informatics and will include discussion of potential policy changes to facilitate effective implementation, adoption, and use of informatics tools in cancer research. An individually authored summary of the workshop will subsequently be prepared by a designated rapporteur.

AGENDA

February 27, 2012

7:30 a.m.   **Breakfast and Registration**

8:00 a.m.   **Welcome from the Institute of Medicine (IOM) National Cancer Policy Forum**
John Mendelsohn, M.D. Anderson Cancer Center
Chair, National Cancer Policy Forum

8:05 a.m.   **Workshop Introduction and Overview**
Sharon Murphy, IOM

SESSION I

Overview of the Informatics Landscape: Where We Are, Framing the Problem, What's Working, What's Not Working, What's Available?
Moderator: Sharon Murphy, IOM

8:15 a.m.   **Challenges, Gaps, and Opportunities in Cancer Informatics**
- Lawrence Shulman, Dana-Farber Cancer Institute

8:30 a.m.	**The Cancer Centers Perspective** • William Dalton, Moffitt Cancer Center & Research Institute
8:50 a.m.	**The Perspective from Cancer Cooperative Group Chairs** • Robert Comis, Eastern Cooperative Oncology Group • Mitchell Schnall, American College of Radiology Imaging Network
9:30 a.m.	**Discussion**
9:45 a.m.	**Coffee Break**
10:00 a.m.	**The Perspective from Clinical Translational Researchers** • Bradley Pollock, University of Texas Health Science Center
10:20 a.m.	**Lessons Learned from caBIG** • Daniel Masys, University of Washington
10:50 a.m.	**Discussion**

KEYNOTE ADDRESS

11:00 a.m.	**Informatics and Personalized Medicine** • Leroy Hood, Institute for Systems Biology
12:00 p.m.	**Lunch Break**

SESSION II

Cancer Use Cases, Examples of Successful Informatics-Supported Endeavors, How Industry Is Addressing Health Care Data, Large-Scale Data Aggregation and Exchange, Overarching Issues, and Reactions
Moderator: Amy Abernethy, Duke University Cancer Care Research Program

1:00 p.m. **DELL-TGen Cloud Computing Collaboration in Personalized Medicine for Pediatric Neuroblastoma**
- August Calhoun, Dell Healthcare and Life Sciences
- Spyro Mousses, TGen

1:30 p.m. **National Comprehensive Cancer Network (NCCN): Database Reporting Systems and Analytics**
- Kimary Kulig, NCCN Clinical and Translational Outcomes Research

2:00 p.m. **Information Technology (IT) Innovations in a Health Care Network Devoted Exclusively to Cancer Research and Treatment**
- Asif Ahmad, Information and Technology Services, US Oncology

2:30 p.m. **Secondary Uses of Data for Comparative Effectiveness Research**
- Paul Wallace, The Lewin Group

3:00 p.m. **Coffee Break**

3:15 p.m. **Panel Discussion**
Moderator: Adam Clark, MedTran Health Strategies

Speakers joined by panelists:
- Gwen Darien, NCI Director's Consumer Liaison Group and cancer survivor
- Deven McGraw, Center for Democracy and Technology
- James Cimino, National Institutes of Health (NIH) Laboratory for Informatics Development
- Steven Piantadosi, Cedars-Sinai Medical Center

4:45 p.m. **Wrap-up**
Amy Abernethy, Duke University Cancer Care Research Program

5:00 p.m. **Adjourn Day 1**

February 28, 2012

7:30 a.m.   **Breakfast and Registration**

SESSION III

Potential Pathways Forward, New Models
Co-moderators: Amy Abernethy, Duke University Cancer Care Research Program, and William Dalton, Moffitt Cancer Center & Research Institute

8:00 a.m.   **Overview of the Needs for Cancer Research**
- John Mendelsohn, M.D. Anderson Cancer Center
  Chair, National Cancer Policy Forum

8:10 a.m.   **Systems and Personalized Medicine Enabled by Public Data**
- Atul Butte, Stanford University School of Medicine

8:55 a.m.   **A Systems-Based Approach to Cancer Informatics**
- George Poste, Arizona State University Complex Adaptive Systems Initiative

9:40 a.m.   **Discussion**

9:50 a.m.   **How Cancer Informatics Will Enable Disruptive Innovation**
- Jason Hwang, Innosight Institute

10:15 a.m.   **Coffee Break**

10:35 a.m.   **Perspectives from the Office of the National Coordinator**
- Farzad Mostashari, Office of the National Coordinator for Health Information Technology

10:55 a.m.   **Electronic Health Records (EHRs) and Cancer Research**
- Sam Butler, Epic

11:05 a.m.	**Democratizing Big Data Informatics for Cancer and Other Therapeutic Areas** • Kris Joshi, Oracle
11:15 a.m.	**Cancer Center–Based Coalitions and IT Networks** • William Dalton, Moffitt Cancer Center & Research Institute
11:35 a.m.	**A Proposal for a Coalition of All Stakeholders to Achieve Data Liquidity in Cancer** • Marcia A. Kean, Feinstein Kean Healthcare
11:50 a.m.	**Panel Discussion** *Moderator:* Lynn Etheredge, Rapid Learning Project, George Washington University Speakers joined by panelists: • Brandon Hayes-Lattin, Oregon Health & Science University and LIVESTRONG • Bradford Hesse, NCI • Mia Levy, Vanderbilt-Ingram Cancer Center • Allen Lichter, American Society of Clinical Oncology
12:50 p.m.	**Summary and Conclusions**
1:00 p.m.	**Adjourn**

Appendix B

Speaker, Moderator, and Panelist Biographies

Amy P. Abernethy, M.D., is a tenured associate professor in the Duke University Schools of Medicine and Nursing, director of the Duke Cancer Care Research Program, and a medical oncologist and palliative medicine physician. She is an appointee to the Institute of Medicine's (IOM's) National Cancer Policy Forum, president-elect of the American Academy of Hospice & Palliative Medicine, a member of the board of directors for the Personalized Medicine Coalition and of the Advisory Board for the Rapid Learning System for Cancer for the American Society of Clinical Oncology, and co-chair of the National Institutes of Health (NIH)–funded Palliative Care Research Cooperative Group. Dr. Abernethy participates integrally in international discussions about reforming the evidence development system, presenting a model for rapid learning health care by coordinating clinical and research functions to better serve patients' needs in an evidence-driven, cost-effective, and patient-centered manner.

Dr. Abernethy is an internationally recognized expert in health services research and delivery in patient-centered cancer care. She directs the Duke Cancer Care Research Program, which conducts patient-centered clinical trials, analyses, and policy studies. The Duke Cancer Care Research Program maintains a large portfolio of NIH, National Cancer Institute (NCI), Agency for Healthcare Research and Quality (AHRQ), philanthropic, and private funding. All studies make use of, and simultaneously contribute to the development of, an integrated data system that coordinates diverse datasets, leverages novel information technology for patient reporting of symptoms and other concerns, informs future studies, and facilitates patient education and patient–provider communication. Dr. Abernethy is co–principal investigator (PI) of the NIH-funded Palliative Care Research Cooperative Group and co-PI of an NCI-funded faculty development (K01) program in comparative effectiveness research to develop the research workforce of the future.

Asif Ahmad, M.B.A., M.S., joined US Oncology, now a part of McKesson Specialty Health, in 2010 as the executive vice president, Technology Services. He currently manages Information and Technology Services, where he is responsible for leading the development and evolution of strategy related to information technology (IT) and the company's several IT-based businesses and services.

Mr. Ahmad served as vice president, Diagnostic Service, and chief information officer and associate dean, Academic Computing and Imaging, School of Medicine at Duke University Health System and Medical Center from 2003 to 2010. Prior to that, he was administrator and chief information officer at the Ohio State University Health System and Medical Center. He earned an M.B.A. at Max M. Fisher College of Business and an M.S. in biomedical engineering at the Ohio State University. He received his B.S. (honors) in electrical engineering from the University of Engineering and Technology in Lahore, Pakistan.

Sam Butler, M.D., brings a wealth of knowledge to Epic's Clinical Informatics Team, with 8 years of senior-level experience in multispecialty medical group management, along with 14 years of clinical practice experience. He helps to guide the direction of Epic's applications. He is heavily involved in the creation and development of Epic and third-party content for use in clinical applications. Dr. Butler has a B.S. in interdisciplinary science and received his M.D. from the University of Florida.

Atul Butte, M.D., Ph.D., is chief of the Division of Systems Medicine and associate professor (tenured) of pediatrics and, by courtesy, medicine and computer science, at Stanford University and Lucile Packard Children's Hospital. Dr. Butte trained in computer science at Brown University, worked as a software engineer at Apple and Microsoft, received his M.D. from Brown University, trained in pediatrics and pediatric endocrinology at Children's Hospital Boston, and received his Ph.D. in health sciences and technology from Harvard Medical School and the Massachusetts Institute of Technology (MIT). He has authored more than 110 publications, delivered more than 120 invited presentations, and received a number of awards, including the Society for Pediatric Research Young Investigator Award, induction into the American College of Medical Informatics, the American Medical Information Association (AMIA) New Investigator Award, the Howard Hughes Medical Institute (HHMI) Early Career Award, and the Pharmaceutical Research and Manufacturers of America (PhRMA) Foundation Research Starter Grant in Informatics. Dr. Butte coauthored one of the first books on microarray analysis, *Microarrays for an Integrative Genomics*, published by MIT Press.

The Butte Laboratory, funded by HHMI and 16 NIH grants, builds and applies tools that convert more than 300 billion points of molecular, clinical, and epidemiological data—measured by researchers and clinicians over the past decade—into diagnostics, therapeutics, and new insights into disease. The Butte Lab has developed tools to index and find genomic datasets based on the phenotypic and contextual details of each experiment, to remap microarray data, to deconvolve multicellular samples, and to perform these calculations on the Internet "cloud." The Butte Lab has used these tools on publicly available molecular data to successfully find new uses for existing drugs and has also been developing novel methods for comparing clinical data from electronic health record (EHR) systems with gene expression data.

August Calhoun, Ph.D., leads the Dell Healthcare and Life Sciences business. The group is responsible for delivering services-based solutions to hospitals, payers, physicians, life sciences companies, and other key players in the health care industry. In this role, Dr. Calhoun oversees global strategy, executive leadership, operations, and business development.

Dr. Calhoun has more than 15 years of experience in the health care and life sciences industry, during which time he has focused on research productivity, life sciences sales force effectiveness, translational medicine, and health care outcomes management. He has expertise in data management, technology strategy, high-performance computing, and process improvement.

Prior to his current role, Dr. Calhoun was responsible for sales and business development of the Dell Healthcare and Life Sciences industry team, where he led efforts to implement innovative solutions to automate operations for health care payers, providers, and life sciences customers.

He has also served Dell customers through end user services optimization, service desk improvement, asset utilization, and remote data center operations.

Prior to joining Dell, Dr. Calhoun worked at the IBM Corporation, where he managed the global pharmaceutical sales and solutions team, as well as a health care consulting team. He was also responsible for relationships with large health care and life sciences clients and held earlier positions in IBM Global Services.

Dr. Calhoun has a Ph.D. in physical chemistry from the University of Pennsylvania in Philadelphia and a B.S. in chemistry from the University of Delaware in Newark.

James Cimino, M.D., is chief of the Laboratory for Informatics Development at the NIH Clinical Center, a senior scientist at the National Library of Medicine (NLM), and an adjunct professor in biomedical informatics at Columbia University. He is charged with the development of an institute-wide Biomedical Translational Research Information System (BTRIS) and conducts clinical informatics research. Dr. Cimino has been an active member of the NLM Board of Scientific Counselors, co-chair of the HL-7 Vocabulary Technical Committee, and a member of the board of the American Medical Informatics Association. He is a fellow of the American College of Medical Informatics, the American College of Physicians, the American Clinical and Climatologic Association, and the New York Academy of Medicine and has received a number of awards.

Previously, Dr. Cimino was with the Center for Medical Informatics (now the Department of Biomedical Informatics) at Columbia University College of Physicians and Surgeons, where he conducted informatics research, built clinical information systems, taught informatics and medicine, and practiced general internal medicine. He published landmark work on controlled terminologies (including a widely adopted set of "desiderata"), the Unified Medical Language System, the use of the Internet in health care, patient access to personal health records, studies of clinician information needs, and development of the "infobutton."

Dr. Cimino received a degree in computers in the biomedical sciences at Brown University and an M.D. at New York Medical College. He completed his medical internship and residency at Saint Vincent's Hospital in New York and an NLM-sponsored research fellowship in medical informatics at Massachusetts General Hospital and the Harvard School of Public Health.

Adam M. Clark, Ph.D., is a patient advocacy consultant and founder, MedTran Health Strategies. Previously, he was a program officer program officer in the Division of Strategic Science and Technology for the Biomedical Advanced Research and Development Authority within the U.S. Department of Health and Human Services (HHS) Office of the Assistant Secretary for Preparedness & Response. In this position he administers drug, diagnostic, and medical technology development programs aimed at advancing medical countermeasures to protect the public health.

Previously, Dr. Clark has worked with numerous patient advocacy and disease research organizations including LIVESTRONG, a cancer research advocacy organization founded by Lance Armstrong, where he served as director of science and health policy. Prior to his work at the foundation, he served as a technology development specialist at NCI, developing programs in cancer biomarker detection technologies. In his time at NCI, Dr. Clark also performed assignments in the White House Office of Science and Technology Policy and the Office of the Secretary of HHS. Dr. Clark has a background in biomedical sciences as a researcher, program administrator, and policy adviser with a focus on molecular diagnostics and personalized medicine.

Dr. Clark has served on several committees and advisory boards, including the Federal Advisory Committee for Health Information Technology Policy at HHS and the NCI Director's Consumer Liaison Group. He earned his Ph.D. from the University of Cincinnati College of Medicine and was trained in science and health policy through the Emerging Leaders Program at HHS.

Robert L. Comis, M.D., is president and chair of the Coalition of Cancer Cooperative Groups (the coalition); group chair of the Eastern Cooperative Oncology Group (ECOG); and professor of medicine and director of the Drexel University Clinical Trials Research Center. A leader in international clinical trials research since 1977, Dr. Comis also serves as president of the ECOG Research and Education Foundation; president of Alpha Oncology, a coalition clinical research division; and chair of ITA Partners.

Dr. Comis is a champion of patient access to cancer clinical trials, spearheading multiple initiatives to raise awareness about the pivotal role of cancer clinical trials in cancer prevention, detection, and treatment. He is a current member of the board of directors for C-Change and the National Coalition for Cancer Research, as well as a past board member of the American Society of Clinical Oncology (ASCO), where he served on a number of

ASCO committees. While chairing the Group Chairs for the Cooperative Group Program, he raised the international profile of the program and initiated efforts to strengthen and reposition it for the future. He has served on a number of editorial boards, authored more than 140 scientific articles, and contributed to more than 20 scientific and medical textbooks on cancer. Dr. Comis is sought as a subject matter expert to the U.S. Congress, the IOM, President's Cancer Panel, National Cancer Advisory Board, and many other national and international organizations.

A graduate of Fordham University, Dr. Comis received his medical degree from the State University of New York (SUNY) Health Science Center School of Medicine, where he also completed his medical internship and residency. He served as a staff associate at NCI and completed a medical oncology fellowship at the Sidney Farber Cancer Center at Harvard Medical School. He has held clinical practice and research leadership positions at Thomas Jefferson University Hospital, Temple University School of Medicine, Fox Chase Cancer Center, and Allegheny Cancer Center. Dr. Comis is a diplomate of the American Board of Internal Medicine and a member of the American College of Physicians–American Society of Internal Medicine.

William S. Dalton, Ph.D., M.D., is CEO of M2Gen, a national biotechnology subsidiary of Moffitt Cancer Center. Until July 2012, Dr. Dalton served as president, CEO, and center director of Moffitt Cancer Center & Research Institute. A nationally renowned cancer researcher, physician, and health policy expert, Dr. Dalton has dedicated his career to the study and development of the most effective approaches to cancer research and care.

Dr. Dalton currently serves as the president of the Association of American Cancer Institutes and is chair of the Science Policy & Legislative Affairs Committee of the American Association for Cancer Research (AACR). In addition, he has served on the NCI Board of Scientific Advisors as well as multiple scientific advisory boards at cancer centers and research foundations.

Dr. Dalton is also interested in the development of personalized cancer care and patient-centered outcomes research. Moffitt's Total Cancer Care is an approach to enhance access to evidence-based, personalized cancer treatments and information or decision tools for patients and clinicians. Total Cancer Care is one of the largest cancer tumor biorepositories and data warehouses in the United States dedicated to use in the development of personalized medicine.

Dr. Dalton received his Ph.D. in toxicology and medical life sciences and his M.D. from Indiana University. He completed his internship in internal medicine at Indiana University and his residency in medicine and fellowships in oncology and clinical pharmacology at the University of Arizona. Prior to accepting the position as CEO and center director at Moffitt, Dr. Dalton was the dean of the College of Medicine at the University of Arizona.

Gwen Darien, a cancer survivor herself, brings a wealth of personal and professional experiences to her position as a director of The Pathways Project, an organization that creates radically inclusive, accessible communities that put people at the center of health care. Ms. Darien served as executive director of the Samuel Waxman Cancer Research Foundation (SWCRF). In this role, she was committed to developing collaborations across all segments of the cancer community to translate cancer research discoveries from the bench to the clinic.

Prior to joining SWCRF, Ms. Darien was editor-in-chief of *CR* magazine and founding director of the American Association for Cancer Research Survivor and Patient Advocacy Program, where she led initiatives to foster mutually beneficial and enduring partnerships among leaders of the cancer survivor, patient advocacy, and scientific communities through collaborations, communications, and education. Ms. Darien was previously the editor-in-chief of *MAMM,* a consumer magazine dedicated to women with breast and reproductive cancer. During Ms. Darien's tenure, *MAMM* won international acclaim for its coverage of survivorship, health disparities, and controversies in women's cancers and health care policy.

Ms. Darien is chair of the NCI Director's Consumer Liaison Group. She is a member of the board of directors of ENACCT (Education Network to Advance Cancer Clinical Trials) and the Strategic Advisory Group (SAGE) of the Center for Patient Partnerships at the University of Wisconsin. She has served on the Secretary's Advisory Committee on Health, Genetics, and Society and the faculties of the AACR-ASCO Methods in Clinical Cancer Research Workshop, the Accelerating Anti-cancer Agent Development and Validation Workshop, and the advisory board of the Health Advocacy Program at Sarah Lawrence College. She has received several awards for her work, including the Avon Foundation Media Leadership Award, the LYMPHAdvocate Award from the Cure for Lymphoma Foundation, and the Sisters' Network Media Leadership Award. She is a graduate of Sarah Lawrence College.

Lynn Etheredge, an independent consultant on health care and social policy issues, works with the Rapid Learning Project at George Washington University. His career started at the White House Office of Management and Budget (OMB). During the Nixon and Ford administrations, he was OMB's principal analyst for Medicare and Medicaid and led its staff work on national health insurance proposals. Mr. Etheredge headed OMB's professional health staff in the Carter and Reagan administrations. Later, he was a coauthor of the Jackson Hole Group's proposals for health care reform and a founding member of the National Academy of Social Insurance. His recent publications include "Medicare's Future: Cancer Care"; "Medicaid: A Future Leader in Effective, High-Quality Care" (an open letter with 12 coauthors); "A Rapid-Learning Health System" (*Health Affairs* special issue); "Administering a Medicaid + Tax Credits Initiative"; and "Technologies of Health Policy." He is author of more than 85 publications and is a graduate of Swarthmore College.

Brandon Hayes-Lattin, M.D., is senior medical adviser for the Lance Armstrong Foundation, an associate professor of medicine in the Division of Hematology and Medical Oncology at Oregon Health & Science University (OHSU), and the director of the OHSU Knight Cancer Institute's Adolescent and Young Adult (AYA) Oncology Program. His clinical background is in the management of hematologic malignancies and the use of hematopoietic stem cell transplantation. However, as a young adult cancer survivor himself and a physician caring for many young adults with hematologic malignancies, Dr. Hayes-Lattin has taken a leadership role in the development of the discipline of adolescent and young adult oncology. He served as the inaugural medical co-chair of the Lance Armstrong Foundation's LIVESTRONG Young Adult Alliance, a coalition of over 150 member organizations leading efforts to research and serve AYA cancer patients. Working in collaboration with the National Cancer Institute, the LIVESTRONG Young Adult Alliance established the Adolescent and Young Adult Oncology Progress Review Group, publishing recommendations and strategic plans for the advancement of AYA Oncology. He currently writes a blog for LIVESTRONG. Dr. Hayes-Lattin also serves on the Expert Advisory Panel to the AYA Committee of the Children's Oncology Group and the Federal Advisory Committee on Breast Cancer in Young Women, and he advises many advocacy groups on the medical needs of cancer patients.

APPENDIX B   *117*

Bradford (Brad) Hesse, Ph.D., is chief of the NCI Health Communication and Informatics Research Branch. For more than two decades, Dr. Hesse has been conducting research in the interdisciplinary fields of social cognition, health communication, health informatics, and user-centered design. He was recruited to NCI in 2003 and has since been focusing on bringing the power of evidence-based health communication technologies to bear on the problem of eliminating death and suffering from cancer. He continues to direct the Health Information National Trends Survey, a biennial general population survey aimed at monitoring the public's use of health information during a period of enhanced capacity at the crest of the information revolution; he also serves as program director for the Centers of Excellence in Cancer Communication Research, a cutting-edge research initiative aimed at expanding the knowledge base underlying effective cancer communication strategies. Dr. Hesse has authored or coauthored more than 150 publications, including peer-reviewed journal articles, technical reports, books, and book chapters. In 2009, his coauthored book entitled *Making Data Talk: Communicating Public Health Data to the Public, Policy Makers, and the Press* was named Book of the Year by the *American Journal of Nursing*.

Dr. Hesse received his degree in social psychology from the University of Utah in 1988 with an accompanying internship in the nascent field of medical informatics and later served as a postdoctoral fellow in the Department of Social and Decision Sciences at Carnegie Mellon University.

Leroy Hood, M.D., Ph.D., is president and co-founder of the Institute for Systems Biology in Seattle. Dr. Hood is a pioneer in systems approaches to biology and medicine. His research has focused on the study of molecular immunology, biotechnology, and genomics. His professional career began at Caltech, where he and his colleagues developed the DNA sequencer and synthesizer and the protein synthesizer and sequencer—four instruments that paved the way for the successful mapping of the human genome and led to his receiving the 2011 prestigious Russ Prize, awarded by the National Academy of Engineering. A pillar in the biotechnology field, Dr. Hood has played a role in founding more than 14 biotechnology companies, including Amgen, Applied Biosystems, Darwin, The Accelerator, and Integrated Diagnostics. He is a member of the National Academy of Sciences, the National Academy of Engineering, and the Institute of Medicine, one of only 15 people in the world to be elected to all three academies. In addition to having published more than 700 peer-reviewed articles, he has coauthored textbooks in biochemistry, immunology, molecular biology, and genetics, as well as a popular book on the human genome project, *The Code of Codes*. He is the recipient of numerous awards, including the Lasker Award, the Kyoto Prize, and the Heinz Award in Technology. Dr. Hood has also received 17 honorary degrees from prestigious universities in the United States and other countries and holds 36 patents.

Jason Hwang, M.D., M.B.A., is an internal medicine physician and cofounder and executive director of Health Care at the Innosight Institute, a nonprofit social innovation think tank based in Mountain View, California. Together with Professor Clayton M. Christensen of Harvard Business School and the late Jerome H. Grossman of the Harvard Kennedy School of Government, he is coauthor of *The Innovator's Prescription: A Disruptive Solution for Health Care*, the American College of Healthcare Executives 2010 Book of the Year, and recipient of the 2011 Health Service Journal Circle Prize for Inspiring Innovation.

Previously, Dr. Hwang taught as chief resident and clinical instructor at the University of California, Irvine, where he received multiple recognitions for his clinical work. He has also served as a clinician with the Southern California Kaiser Permanente Medical Group and the Department of Veterans Affairs Medical Center in Long Beach, California. Dr. Hwang received his B.S. and M.D. from the University of Michigan and his M.B.A. from Harvard Business School.

Kris Joshi, Ph.D., is global vice president for Oracle's health care product portfolio. Dr. Joshi helped launch the Health Sciences Global Business Unit within Oracle, and in his prior role as head of Strategy and Operations, he led the business unit's growth strategy, including the acquisitions of Relsys and Phase Forward. He oversees a broad product portfolio that covers analytics, health information exchange, care management, and "convergence" solutions for personalized medicine and translational research that serve both health care and life sciences customers.

Dr. Joshi brings deep experience across business and technology strategy, M&A, operations, sales, marketing, and business transformation. Prior to Oracle, he served in senior strategy roles in IBM's Global Sales and Distribution Organization, where he helped shape IBM's global distribution and emerging markets strategies. Prior to IBM, Dr. Joshi spent several years as a consultant with McKinsey and Company, where he served Fortune 500 clients in the banking, media, health care, and life sciences industries on business strategy issues.

Dr. Joshi has a long-standing personal commitment to help bridge the gap between the social and business worlds through entrepreneurship, innovation, and public–private partnerships. He has championed numerous initiatives aimed at leveraging technology to improve the quality, safety, and affordability of health care globally.

Dr. Joshi holds a B.S. in mathematics from Caltech and a Ph.D. in astrophysics from MIT.

Marcia Kean, M.B.A., has built Feinstein Kean Healthcare's national role in the life sciences since the firm's inception 25 years ago. She served as the CEO of the firm from 2002 to 2011 and became chair of Strategic Initiatives in 2011.

Ms. Kean has more than 35 years of biomedical industry experience, in support of hundreds of start-ups and publicly traded companies, as well as large-scale national and international science and technology-driven programs. She has decades of business operating experience as well as knowledge of the development and implementation of public–private projects undertaken by multistakeholder ecosystems.

In 2003, Ms. Kean founded the first molecular medicine communications practice in the country. She has served as an adviser to the Personalized Medicine Coalition (PMC) since its inception and was awarded that organization's first Distinguished Service Award in 2006. She has served on the planning committee for the Harvard–Partners Center for Personalized Genetic Medicine annual personalized medicine conference since its inception. She served in 2006 as a member of the Personalized Health Care Expert Panel convened by the Office of the Assistant Secretary for Planning and Evaluation (ASPE) of HHS. She chairs the Advisory Committee of Turning the Tide Against Cancer Through Sustained Medical Innovation, a national conference on science and policy co-hosted by the Personalized Medicine Coalition, American Association for Cancer Research, and Feinstein Kean Healthcare.

Ms. Kean holds an M.B.A. in finance from New York University and a B.A. from the University of California, Berkeley.

Kimary Kulig, Ph.D., M.P.H., is vice president of clinical and translational outcomes research at the National Comprehensive Cancer Network (NCCN). Her primary responsibility is to direct the ongoing development and advancement of the NCCN Oncology Outcomes Database (NCCN Database) and other outcomes research programs. The NCCN Database is a set of databases with comprehensive data, including clinical outcomes, on five major tumor types for thousands of patients treated at NCCN member institutions.

Prior to joining NCCN, Dr. Kulig worked for several years leading outcomes-based research in oncology at Pfizer, Inc., most recently as senior director and lead, Molecular Epidemiology Research, Oncology. In this role, she designed and conducted biomarker-linked outcomes research projects in support of multiple clinical development programs, including those involving companion diagnostics, at the global level.

Prior to Dr. Kulig's appointment at Pfizer, Inc., she led an epidemiology and surveillance research program for the Arthritis Foundation, conducted public health research at the Columbia University Mailman School of Public Health and the Centers for Disease Control and Prevention, and engaged in immunology research at Columbia University's College of Physicians and Surgeons, the Kennedy Institute of Rheumatology (London), and the Mayo Clinic (Rochester, Minnesota).

Dr. Kulig holds a master's degree in public health with an emphasis in epidemiology from the Columbia University Mailman School of Public Health and earned her doctorate in immunology and molecular oncology from the New York University School of Medicine.

Mia A. Levy, M.D., Ph.D., is director of cancer clinical informatics for the Vanderbilt-Ingram Cancer Center and assistant professor of biomedical informatics and medicine. Dr. Levy received her undergraduate degree in bioengineering from the University of Pennsylvania in 1997 and her medical doctorate from Rush University in 2003. She then spent six years at Stanford University for postgraduate training in internal medicine and medical oncology while completing her Ph.D. in biomedical informatics. She joined the faculty at Vanderbilt as an assistant professor of biomedical informatics and medicine in August 2009. She is a practicing medical oncologist specializing in the treatment of breast cancer.

Dr. Levy's research interests include biomedical informatics methods to support the continuum of cancer care and cancer research. Current research projects include informatics methods for (1) image-based cancer treatment response assessment using quantitative imaging, (2) clinical decision support for treatment prioritization of molecular subtypes of cancer, (3) protocol-based plan management, and (4) learning cancer systems.

Allen S. Lichter, M.D., is CEO of ASCO, the world's leading professional organization, representing nearly 30,000 physicians and health professionals in oncology.

Prior to joining ASCO in 2006, Dr. Lichter was at the University of Michigan in two significant leadership roles. He served as chair and professor of radiation oncology from 1984 to 1998 and as dean of the Medical School from 1998 to 2006. Dr. Lichter was named the first Isadore Lampe Professor of Radiation Oncology, an endowed chair, and also was the Newman Family Professor of Radiation Oncology.

Prior to his tenure at the University of Michigan, Dr. Lichter was director of the Radiation Therapy Section of NCI's Radiation Oncology Branch. Dr. Lichter's research and development of three-dimensional treatment planning led to a Gold Medal from the American Society for Therapeutic Radiology and Oncology. In 2002, he was elected to the Institute of Medicine of the National Academies of Sciences.

As a member of ASCO since 1980, Dr. Lichter has assumed many prominent roles in the Society, including president (1998–1999) and founding chair of ASCO's Conquer Cancer Foundation Board.

Dr. Lichter earned a bachelor's degree (1968) and a medical degree (1972) from the University of Michigan. He trained in radiation oncology at the University of California, San Francisco, before joining the faculty at Johns Hopkins University and later NCI.

Daniel R. Masys, M.D., is affiliate professor of biomedical and health informatics at the University of Washington (UW), Seattle. An honors graduate of Princeton University and the Ohio State University College of Medicine, he completed postgraduate training in internal medicine, hematology, and medical oncology at the University of California, San Diego, and the Naval Regional Medical Center, San Diego. His more than 30-year career in biomedical informatics prior to joining UW included leadership positions at NCI and NLM and faculty appointments at the University of California, San Diego, and the Vanderbilt University School of Medicine, where he was emeritus professor and chair of the Department of Biomedical Informatics.

Dr. Masys is an elected member of the Institute of Medicine. He is a fellow of the American College of Physicians and a fellow and past president of the American College of Medical Informatics. He was a founding associate editor of the *Journal of the American Medical Informatics Association* and has received numerous awards including the NIH Director's Award and the U.S. Surgeon General's Exemplary Service Medal.

Deven McGraw, J.D., L.L.M., is director of the Health Privacy Project at the Center for Democracy and Technology (CDT). The project is focused on developing and promoting workable privacy and security protections for electronic personal health information.

Ms. McGraw is active in efforts to advance the adoption and implementation of health information technology and electronic health information exchange to improve health care. She was one of three people appointed by Kathleen Sebelius, secretary of HHS, to serve on the Health Information Technology (HIT) Policy Committee, a federal advisory committee established in the American Recovery and Reinvestment Act of 2009. She chairs the Committee's Privacy and Security Workgroup (the "Tiger Team") and serves as a member of its Meaningful Use and Information Exchange Workgroups. She also served on the Policy Steering Committee of the eHealth Initiative and now serves on its Leadership Council. She is also on the Steering Group of the Markle Foundation's Connecting for Health multistakeholder initiative.

Ms. McGraw has a strong background in health care policy. Prior to joining CDT, she was the chief operating officer of the National Partnership for Women & Families, providing strategic direction and oversight for all of the organization's core program areas, including the promotion of initiatives to improve health care quality. Ms. McGraw also was an associate in the public policy group at Patton Boggs, LLP and in the health care group at Ropes & Gray. She served as deputy legal counsel to the governor of Massachusetts and taught in the Federal Legislation Clinic at Georgetown University Law Center.

Ms. McGraw graduated magna cum laude from the University of Maryland. She earned her J.D., magna cum laude, and her L.L.M. from Georgetown University Law Center and was executive editor of the *Georgetown Law Journal.* She also has a master of public health degree from the Johns Hopkins Bloomberg School of Hygiene and Public Health.

John Mendelsohn, M.D., was president of the University of Texas M.D. Anderson Cancer Center in Houston from 1996 until 2011. Under his direction, M.D. Anderson assumed a leadership role in translational and clinical cancer research and was named the top cancer hospital in the United States for 8 of the past 10 years in the *U.S. News & World Report* "America's

Best Hospitals" survey. Currently, Dr. Mendelsohn is the co-director of the Khalifa Institute for Personalized Cancer Therapy at M.D. Anderson. Previously, he chaired the Department of Medicine at Memorial Sloan-Kettering Cancer Center, and he began his career at the University of California, San Diego (UCSD), in La Jolla, where he was founding director of its cancer center. Dr. Mendelsohn and his collaborators pioneered the concept of therapy to target the products of genes that cause cancer. His team's innovative research on inhibition of the epidermal growth factor (EGF) receptor tyrosine kinase led to production and investigation of monoclonal antibody C225 (Erbitux), which is approved by the Food and Drug Administration (FDA) for colon cancer and head and neck cancer. He served as founding editor-in-chief of *Clinical Cancer Research,* has published more than 250 articles and reviews, and has received many prizes and awards. Dr. Mendelsohn is chair of the IOM's National Cancer Policy Forum. He has directed postdoctoral programs that trained many dozens of medical oncologists and scientists. He is an active board member of several Houston area organizations, including the Houston Grand Opera, the BioHouston, and the Center for Houston's Future.

Farzad Mostashari, M.D., Sc.M., is national coordinator for health information technology within the Office of the National Coordinator for Health Information Technology (ONC) at HHS. Farzad joined ONC in July 2009. Previously, he served at the New York City Department of Health and Mental Hygiene as assistant commissioner for the Primary Care Information Project, where he facilitated the adoption of prevention-oriented health information technology by more than 1,500 providers in underserved communities. Dr. Mostashari also led the Centers for Disease Control and Prevention (CDC)–funded New York City Center of Excellence in Public Health Informatics and an AHRQ-funded project focused on quality measurement at the point of care. Prior to this, he established the Bureau of Epidemiology Services at the New York City Department of Health, charged with providing epidemiologic and statistical expertise and data for decision making to the health department.

He completed his graduate training at the Harvard School of Public Health and Yale Medical School, his internal medicine residency at Massachusetts General Hospital, and completed the CDC's Epidemic Intelligence Service. He was one of the lead investigators in the outbreaks of West Nile virus and anthrax in New York City and was among the first developers of real-time electronic disease surveillance systems nationwide.

Spyro Mousses, Ph.D., is professor at the Translational Genomics Research Institute (TGen), in Phoenix, Arizona. His scientific background and expertise include developing platform genomic and computational technologies and he recently has focused on strategically integrating multiple technologies and scientific resources to engineer innovative solutions that can support drug discovery, translational research, clinical drug development, and personalized medicine. Toward the goal of integrating technologies across sectors into unifying solutions, Dr. Mousses has lead multidisciplinary public–private collaborations and developed partnerships with major corporations in the pharmaceutical, biotech, life sciences, and IT industries. He is also a mission-driven entrepreneur and has served as chief scientific officer and co-founder of Systems Medicine Inc. (acquired by Cell Therapeutics Inc.) and MedTrust OnLine Inc. (acquired by Annai Systems Inc.). Dr. Mousses received his B.Sc. (pharmacology and toxicology), M.Sc., and Ph.D. (molecular pathogenesis and genetics of cancer) from the University of Toronto. He served as staff scientist at the National Human Genome Research Institute, NIH, where he led a program in cancer genome scanning and high-throughput technology development. He joined TGen at its inception as one of the founding scientists, contributing to building and directing the Cancer Drug Development Laboratory and the Pharmaceutical Genomics Division. Most recently, he was appointed director of the Center for BioIntelligence and was named vice president in the Office of Innovation.

Sharon Murphy, M.D., joined the Institute of Medicine as a scholar-in-residence in October 2008, coming to the District of Columbia from Texas, where she was inaugural director of the Greehey Children's Cancer Research Institute and professor of pediatrics at the University of Texas Health Science Center at San Antonio from 2002 to 2008.

From 1988 to 2002, Dr. Murphy was chief of the Division of Hematology-Oncology at Children's Memorial Hospital in Chicago and professor of pediatrics at Northwestern University School of Medicine, where she also led the program in pediatric oncology at the Robert H. Lurie Cancer Center. From 1974 to 1988, Dr. Murphy was on the faculty at St. Jude Children's Research Hospital in Memphis.

A pediatric oncologist and clinical cancer researcher, Dr. Murphy has devoted the past 35 years to improving cure rates for childhood cancer, particularly childhood lymphomas and leukemias. She was chair of the Pediatric Oncology Group from 1993 to 2001. She has been recognized for her achievements by the Association of Community Cancer Centers (2001), the Distinguished Service Award for Scientific Leadership from ASCO (2005), and the Distinguished Career Award from the American Society of Pediatric Hematology and Oncology (2009).

The author of more than 220 original articles, reviews, and book chapters, Dr. Murphy has also served on numerous editorial boards. She has been a member of the boards of directors of the American Cancer Society, AACR, the American Society of Hematology, and ASCO, and she has been an adviser to NCI and FDA.

She earned her bachelor of science degree from the University of Wisconsin (1965) and her medical degree, cum laude, from Harvard Medical School (1969). She completed postdoctoral training in pediatrics at the University of Colorado (1969–1971) and in pediatric hematology and oncology at the University of Pennsylvania (1971–1973).

Steven Piantadosi, M.D., Ph.D., is director of the Samuel Oschin Comprehensive Cancer Institute at Cedars-Sinai Medical Center. Dr. Piantadosi's role is to lead the medical center's programs in cancer research, treatment, and education; enhance academic activities related to cancer; and bring together Cedars-Sinai's cancer physicians and researchers for innovative collaborations.

Prior to joining Cedars-Sinai in December 2007, Dr. Piantadosi was professor of oncology at the Johns Hopkins University School of Medicine and director of biostatistics at the Sidney Kimmel Comprehensive Cancer Center. He also was a professor of biostatistics and of epidemiology at the Bloomberg School of Public Health. After earning his medical degree from the University of North Carolina and his doctorate in biomathematics from the University of Alabama at Birmingham, Dr. Piantadosi became a senior staff fellow at NCI.

Dr. Piantadosi is one of the world's leading experts in the design and analysis of clinical trials for cancer research. In addition to advising both FDA and industry, he has served on external advisory boards for NIH and other prominent cancer programs and centers.

The author of more than 230 peer-reviewed scientific articles, Dr. Piantadosi has published extensively on research results, clinical applications, and trial methodology. While his papers have contributed to many diverse areas of oncology, he has also collaborated on studies in disciplines outside cancer including lung disease, AIDS, and degenerative neurological disease. Dr. Piantadosi is the author of *Clinical Trials: A Methodologic*

Perspective, which is widely considered a classic textbook for clinical trials. He has taught young investigators extensively in his own course, the University of California, Los Angeles (UCLA), STAR program, and through international venues such as the AACR-ASCO Workshop on Methods in Clinical Cancer Research. Dr. Piantadosi has held leadership roles with national cooperative oncology groups and has been a member of numerous clinical trial monitoring committees.

Bradley H. Pollock, M.P.H., Ph.D., is professor and the founding chair of the Department of Epidemiology and Biostatistics in the School of Medicine at the University of Texas Health Science Center at San Antonio (UTHSCSA). He holds adjunct professorships at the University of Texas School of Public Health, the College of Business at the University of Texas at San Antonio, and the Department of Statistics at Texas A&M University. In 2001, he started the Center for Epidemiology and Biostatistics at UTHSCSA, which evolved into the Department of Epidemiology and Biostatistics in 2006.

Dr. Pollock served as a cooperative group statistician for the Pediatric Oncology Group (POG) and the successor Children's Oncology Group (COG). He has been responsible for the biostatistical management of Phase I through Phase III cancer clinical trials, correlative biology studies, interventional trials, and numerous observational studies. He has served continuously as principal investigator of the Community Clinical Oncology Program (CCOP) Research Base grant for POG and COG since 1995, chair of the POG Epidemiology Committee from 1991 to 2000, and chair of the POG and COG Cancer Control Committees from 1995 to 2003.

Dr. Pollock serves as director of the Biostatistics and Informatics Shared Resource for the P30-funded NCI-designated Cancer Therapy & Research Center (CTRC). He also directs two cores for the NIH-funded Clinical & Translational Science Award (CTSA) at UTHSCSA: the Biostatistics, Epidemiology, and Research Design Core and the Biomedical Informatics Core. Dr. Pollock is the current vice chair and chair-elect of the CTSA Biostatistics/Epidemiology/Research Design Key Function Committee. In addition, he is president of the Association of Clinical Translational Statisticians.

Dr. Pollock's research focuses on pediatric and adolescent oncology, with an emphasis on cancer epidemiology and cancer prevention and control research. He has served on numerous NIH grant review and other scientific committees.

Dr. Pollock received his B.S. in biological sciences from the University of California, Irvine, and his M.P.H. and Ph.D. in epidemiology (minor in biostatistics) from the UCLA School of Public Health.

George Poste, Ph.D., D.V.M., is chief scientist for the Complex Adaptive Systems Initiative (http://www.casi.asu.edu) at Arizona State University (ASU). From 2003 to 2009, he created and built the Biodesign Institute at ASU (http://www.biodesign.asu.edu).

He serves on the board of directors of Monsanto, Exelixis, and Caris Life Sciences and the scientific advisory board of Synthetic Genomics. From 1992 to 1999, he was chief science and technology officer of SmithKline Beecham. In 2004 he was named R&D Scientist of the Year by *R&D Magazine*; in 2006, he received the Einstein award from the Global Business Leadership Council; and in 2009, he received the Scrip Lifetime Achievement award.

Dr. Poste is a fellow of the Royal Society (UK), the Royal College of Pathologists, and the Academy of Medical Sciences (UK); a distinguished fellow at the Hoover Institution, Stanford University; and a member of the Council for Foreign Relations and the IOM Forum on Microbial Threats.

Mitchell D. Schnall, M.D., Ph.D., is an international leader in translational biomedical and imaging research, working throughout his career across the interface between basic imaging science and clinical medicine to ensure effective integration of radiology research with other medical disciplines. His work has led to fundamental changes in the imaging approaches to breast and prostate cancer, and he continues to have a significant influence on emerging imaging technologies, including those in optical imaging.

Dr. Schnall was elected group chair of the American College of Radiology Imaging Network (ACRIN) in 2008, after having served as its deputy chair from 1999 through 2007. ACRIN is an NCI-sponsored cancer cooperative group that designs, conducts, and reports on multicenter clinical trials of imaging in cancer and conducts similar research in neurology and cardiovascular studies through non-NCI funding. Among the multiple ACRIN clinical studies under Dr. Schnall's direction are the National Lung Screening Trial, the Digital Mammography Imaging Screening Trial, and the National CT (computed tomography) Colonography Trial. Dr. Schnall is co-PI of the Center for Magnetic Resonance and Optical Imaging, an NIH-funded regional resource at the University of Pennsylvania.

Dr. Schnall maintains active membership in the American Society for

Clinical Investigation, the Association of American Physicians, ASCO, and the Radiological Society of North America. He received his undergraduate, medical, and doctoral degrees from the University of Pennsylvania, where he has served on the faculty of the Radiology Department since 1991 and as full professor since 2002.

Lawrence N. Shulman, M.D., is chief medical officer, senior vice president for medical affairs, and chief, Division of General Oncology, Department of Medical Oncology, at Dana-Farber Cancer Institute (DFCI). He focuses his efforts on clinical services for both adult and pediatric care at DCFI and its partners, Brigham and Women's Hospital and Children's Hospital.

Dr. Shulman has served as one of the component leaders through the DFCI strategic planning initiative. He is director of network development for Dana-Farber–Brigham and Women's Cancer Center and oversees DFCI ambulatory oncology units at several regional sites. He is also physician leader for the development of clinical information systems for DFCI. He is chair of the ASCO Quality of Care Committee and a member of ASCO's Health Information Technology Workgroup. He is also a member of the ASCO Workgroup on Provider-Payer Initiatives. He is a member of the Commission on Cancer of the American College of Surgeons and vice chair of its Quality Integration Committee.

A specialist in the treatment of patients with breast cancer, his research includes the development of new cancer therapies. He works closely with Partners in Health, where he is senior adviser in oncology, helping to lead the development of a structured cancer program for its resource-limited health care sites in Rwanda, Malawi, and Haiti. He was the founding co-chair, together with Dr. Julio Frenk, dean of the Harvard School of Public Health, of the Global Task Force on Expanding Access to Cancer Care and Control in the Developing World, a Harvard-based, international task force committed to the improvement of cancer care worldwide.

PauPaul J. Wallace, M.D., is senior vice president and director, Center for Comparative Effectiveness Research at The Lewin Group. Dr. Wallace is a board-certified physician in internal medicine and hematology and a researcher and lecturer on topics relating to comparative effectiveness research (CER), including evidence-based medicine practice and policy, performance improvement and measurement, clinical practice guideline development; population-based care and disease management, new technology assessment, and comparative assessment.

He has participated on several IOM advisory committees; he currently serves as a member of the Board on Population Health and Public Health Practice, and he chaired the committee that produced the recent report *Primary Care and Public Health: Exploring Integration to Improve Population Health*. He is vice chair of the board of directors for AcademyHealth and a board member of the eHealth Initiative.

Dr. Wallace previously served on the National Advisory Committee for AHRQ; the Medical Coverage Advisory Committee, Center for Medicare and Medicaid Services (CMS); and the Committee on Performance Measurement for the National Committee on Quality Assurance (NCQA). Before joining The Lewin Group in 2011, he was medical director for health and productivity management programs at Kaiser Permanente's national Permanente Federation. He had served as a physician and administrator with Kaiser for more than 20 years. Prior to his work at Kaiser, he taught clinical and basic sciences and investigated bone marrow function as a faculty member at the Oregon Health Sciences University.

Dr. Wallace is a graduate of the University of Iowa School of Medicine and completed further training in internal medicine, hematology, and cancer research at Strong Memorial Hospital and the University of Rochester.